The Ecology of Gentle Birth

BY ROBIN LIM

For Debra
Terima kasih
Maraming Salamat po
Thank you ♡
for your Devotion
MOMS & Babies... &
families.
love
Ibu Robin

Half Angel Press

Half Angel Press
P.O. Box 116, Ubud
Bali, Indonesia - 80571

Illustrations by Loretta Viscuso
Cover photo 'Lakota and Rimba' by Robin Lim
Cover typesetting by David Blyth
Cover design by Zion Lee
Book design by Lakota Moira
Edited by Wil Hemmerle

Illustrations on page 76-79 by Gede Robi Supriyanto

Illustrations on page 171-177 by Marcia Barnett-Lopez

Illustrations on page 213 by Zion Lee

First printing 2016
Printed in the United States

ISBN: 0-9762907-6-6

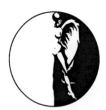 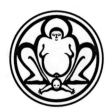 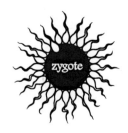

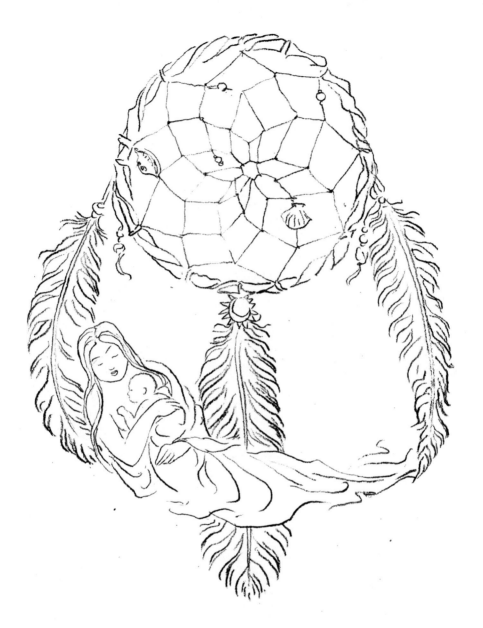

All the Mothers in my line, the Grandmothers
and Great-great-grandmothers, had the innate wisdom to grow healthy,
strong, intelligent babies. Their blood flows through my body,
they passed to me their deep-rooted intuitive instinctive blessings,
this pregnancy now, is proof of their lifetimes of love.

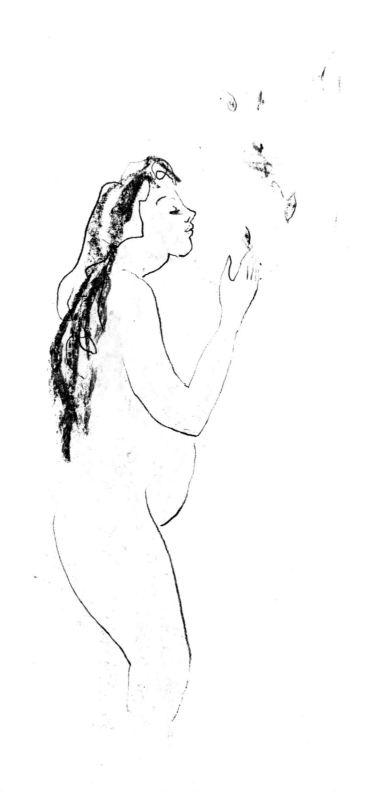

Contents

Introduction

by Deborah Flowers, Farm Midwife

My first birth was the most empowering experience of my life! After my son was born I felt like I could whip the world with one hand tied behind my back. This is what birth should be like for all women. You need to feel empowered as you enter motherhood. The information in this book can help you to prepare for your best possible birth experience.

It is a good thing that pregnancy is nine months long, it gives you time to prepare mentally, physically, and spiritually. Some women seem to think that there is nothing that they can do. Their body grows the baby without instruction from them and then the doctor or midwife "delivers" the baby and it is all out of their control. You would not go to the Olympics without preparing. Or act in a play without rehearsing. There are lots of things that you can be doing during your pregnancy to prepare.

I am a big believer in the philosophy that "prevention is better than a cure". There are many things that you can be doing during your pregnancy to help prevent problems. In my home birth practice I often spend 2-3 hours with women at each prenatal visit teaching and answering questions. Reading this book is like having prenatal visits with Ibu Robin.

I agree with Ibu Robin that it is important to find care providers whose beliefs are as much in alignment with your own as you can in order to have the best possible birth experience. If you are not able to find a midwife where you live, find a Doctor who is the most like-minded that you can, and hire a Doula (a non-medical care giver trained to mother the mother).

Read books with wonderful birth stories. If someone comes up to you and tries to tell you horror stories about birth, then very sweetly say to them, "Oh, didn't you know, you are not supposed to tell pregnant women anything but good stories about birth." Then walk away. After your birth tell good stories to the pregnant women you meet and to your daughters. This was the best gift that my mother gave me. She told me not to believe women who told me that birth hurt. She said it was not that bad and that I could do it. I believed what my mother told me because I knew she was wise.

It is up to women to make changes in how our babies are born. Educate yourself and let your care providers know what you want. Seek out like-minded care providers. You have the power to make a difference for yourself and all women.

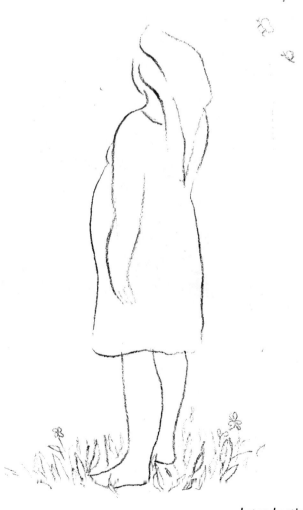

Forward

We live in the epoch of Climate Change, which threatens the very Earthly home of each and every individual, of every species. Why then do we still have children? Perhaps imbedded in our DNA is a belief that each new baby is a promise that the world will survive. That people, as the dominant species, will become parents, and in that process, open their hearts, minds and deeds, to innovate and implement real solutions to the world's myriad of problems. Each individual really can make a difference. Hence, the "Ecology of Gentle Mothering." I believe that world peace, and environmental security begins in the womb and is nurtured at the breasts of women. Welcome to Mothering, the most essential significant important job on the planet.

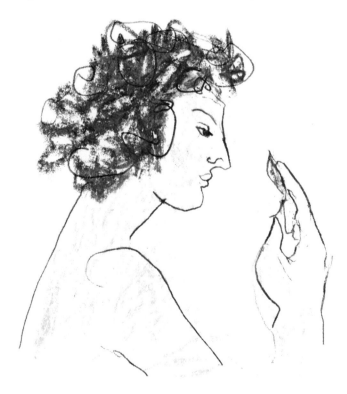

I am quite convinced that nothing tests our humanity like bringing a newborn human Earth-side. It is necessary to become a heroine to become a mother. Pregnancy and childbirth, postpartum, breastfeeding and mothering are outstanding achievements. Being a mom is a superpower. Yet, it is the softest most open-hearted, sacred feminine endeavor in the world. Motherhood is the loveliest conundrum.

Each of us wears masks and builds layers of protection. We survive in the harsh hive of society due to our cunning at hiding and shielding our authentic selves from any perceived threat. This begins at birth, if there is trauma. It grows as childhood unfolds, with the first criticisms and embarrassments we experience. Over the course of our lifetime we grow a persona and wear it day and night, like a well fitting mask, until we perceive this "animus" persona made to survive in a 'masculine' world of business and survival, as our true self.

Physically your pregnancy may be amazing, beautiful and challenging, all at once. Labor is an intricate dance of hormones and DNA memories, all that you are made of and all that your cells have learned. This organized whole, YOU, draws the map that guides your process of contractions, the cervix opening, and the body yielding so the baby may descend into the Star Gate of your pelvis, pass through the birth canal and emerge, alive and full of wonder. Psychologically and spiritually labor is the process of removing masks and stripping away each and every layer of protection we have manufactured over a lifetime. Labor and birth are driven by a cocktail of hormones, predominantly the very shy hormone oxytocin, hormone of love. Only the oxytocin rich core of our being, naked and vulnerable, soft, surrendered, strong, determined and unburnished, may give birth naturally.

The more reinforced and defended one is, the longer and more challenging labor may be. And, that's ok too. There is no one-size-fits-all road to motherhood. We humans have learned through traumas, large and small, to hold-on to our layers of protection. Yet, only by letting go to do we cross the bridge into motherhood. In our complicated day and age, women coping with perceived and real threats may face childbirth charged with fear. However, women are so much stronger and more determined than any fears.

Over the ages BirthKeepers (midwives, nurses, doctors, doulas, mothers, grandmothers, and families) have learned, how to weave a web of safety around the expectant mother, so that she may let-go and give birth.

The soaring rate of technology in childbirth, augmented and instrumental birth, cesarean birth, anesthesia for childbirth, are all modern solutions to the 'problem' of women having difficulty feeling safe enough to let-go and let birth unfold. This 'problem' in many cases, is created by the procedures, personnel and place, where the birth is happening. Obstacles in childbirth are all too often the effect of oxytocin, the very shy hormone of love, being unable to flow. Today more and more women are delivered of their babies, by force, because their process of birthing is considered too long, or is deemed obstructed. It takes time and patience to un-build the fortress of our animus. The gentle process of unwinding and birthing, is perceived, by some medical professionals, who endeavor to protect us, (and yes, make money from us) as "too risky." In technological environments, charged with fear, natural childbirth is becoming more and more rare and endangered.

For the small percentage of MotherBabies who really need cesarean birth, I applaud your courage. Well done, brave mother. Wisely used, when truly needed, cesarean birth saves lives. If you had a cesarean birth you feel was unnecessary, love is the healing answer, the only answer. No one should be made to feel she failed or is inadequate, because her baby was born via cesarean birth. She DID give birth. Perhaps it was not the birth a particular mother dreamed of and planned… yet, it was a birth, a miracle.

Natural childbirth is not a myth, most women CAN do it, supported by loving skilled BirthKeepers (Midwives, Doctors, Doulas, Nurses & caring family). I am not saying there are easy answers or simple solutions. I am saying that as a mother-to-be, you must touch in with your INNER KNOWING, in this journey toward motherhood. When you find her, your authentic self, it will not matter how your birth unfolds, for it will be just right, for you and for your baby.

You may perceive challenges, and let them go. You can do it if you are a first time mom, or an experienced mother. With support, you can do it if you have had previous cesarean birth.

The first step is to acknowledge your fears surrounding pregnancy, labor and childbirth and release them. Un-build your fortress personality, and layer-by-layer, you will reveal your authentic self. Your authentic self is so loving and kind. This is the YOU your baby has chosen as his or her mother.

Prenatal care, is NOT intended to be "prenatal scare." Search for a midwife and/or a doctor who will become your partners-in-health, by sharing knowledge, and supporting your feeling of safety. Surround yourself with friends, family and healthcare providers who BELIEVE in you. As you enliven your inner knowing, most pregnancy discomforts can be resolved and released, and your health will soar. This little book was written to help you un-build the fortress, and let down your guard so you may allow your oxytocin to flow. Prepare your heart to arrive for your childbirth experience, dressed in your authentic self, ready to open and become a mother, as nature intended it.

By consciously bringing your baby Earth-side, you are taking a giant leap, toward healing MotherEarth, bless you.

~ Ibu Robin Lim
August 2014 from 27,000 ft. flying above the Philippines
& Christmas Eve 2015, flying from Bali to Costa Rica to receive a baby

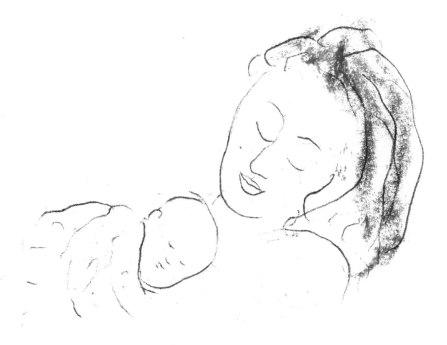

"What if more women, mothers, gave birth as an ecstatic celebration of female sexuality? Mothers who do will often declare, "Now I can do anything!" What would the world look like if half of our population felt empowered to make a difference with their lives?"

~ Jeannine Parvati

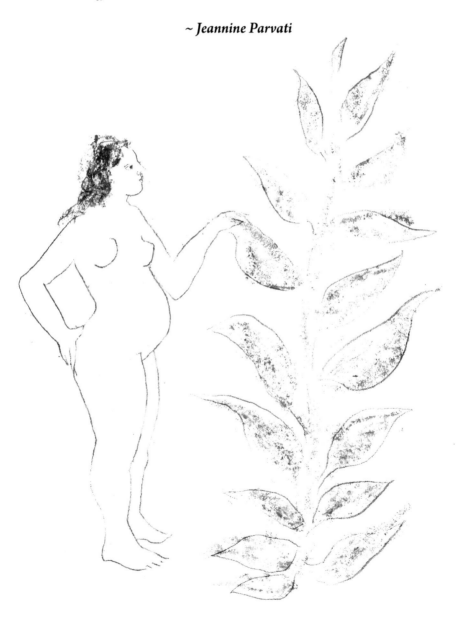

Harmony with Nature

This book is made to inspire you as a woman emerging into motherhood, to become a wise-woman. It is meant to help you enliven your own DIVINE INNER KNOWING. BirthKeepers, Midwives, Doulas, open-hearted Doctors, Nurses and Families must learn to support the most natural approach to motherhood, as it empowers the woman and helps her recognize her value as a person, a mother, and an essential part of society. In addition, the more naturally you can live, while pregnant, during labor, and in childbirth, while postpartum and breastfeeding, the healthier you and your baby shall be. Each healthy mother contributes to the health of MotherEarth. Making a small footprint on our Earth is a goal worthy of striving for. Our planet is ailing, and we need to protect her, if your baby and all children are to have a home in the future. Every bit of technology has a price, ecologically. Your choices make a difference for the survival of the planet. Even how you will diaper your baby, with cloth, or with 'disposable' diapers, will profoundly impact our world. Throw-away diapers are not truly 'disposable,' for they do not biodegrade and are a big burden for our environment.

Choosing the natural way in pregnancy and childbirth helps you to respect the power of Mother Nature, Father Time and Love... at work in your body. Conception, the growth of baby in your womb, birth, postpartum, breastfeeding and parenting, are the sacred spiral of reproduction. This gift, and life force, work best if we are in harmony with nature.

Harmony for a pregnant woman means that she and her family support her health and provide for all the needs of the new baby growing within. To be healthy and to have a healthy baby, pregnant women need to breathe clean air, drink pure water, and eat natural healthy foods. Love is the secret ingredient that helps our cells absorb all the nutrients. Literally, some people are starving for love, just as our Earth Mother is starving for care.

Expectant mothers must find a balance between gentle exercise, activities like work, play, worship and rest. Pregnant women dream of having a healthy, happy, intelligent and creative child. This book is dedicated to that dream, because, healthy mothers are more likely to have healthy babies. A healthy planet is necessary, so that our babies, our children, may have a home.

**Tsaraki (Cherokee) Blessing
for the Newborn Human:**

*"May you live long enough
to know why you were born."*

Does JOY have a function in making healthy babies?

YES!

Most profoundly, pregnant women, promised mothers, need love, happiness, and nurturing. Cortisol is a slow-acting hormone that scientists have been studying in pregnancy. When a person is depressed, anxious, bereaved, under stress or unhappy, higher levels of cortisol will be found in her body. It is well understood that cortisol inhibits fetal growth and activity, even impairing brain development in the baby. Your baby's health and intelligence are significantly affected by your emotional state during pregnancy. I like to tell the young fathers-to-be (or partner of the mother ~ not all families look alike), "If you want a healthy, happy, smart baby: make your partner laugh. Happiness is indeed medicine for the soul and it helps developing babies grow strong in body, mind and spirit.

When I was expecting my 4th baby, I was a single mother. Life as I knew it was melting down, and I was painfully aware of how the sorrow I was experiencing could affect my developing baby. I made a conscious choice, to enjoy the happy moments, the snapshots of joy. I hoped that by focusing on these moments and allowing them to glow, I could perhaps override the stress and sadness. I found that by not trying to solve all my problems at once, I could enjoy the tiny moments of pleasure. I would smile, and even laugh. I felt delight when my small daughter used new words, or my son stopped to rescue an earthworm. There was bliss when my eldest helped me to plant the vegetable garden. I found refuge in the hugs my midwife gave me, saying, "You got a lot of good coming." Had I focused on unhappiness, I would have been too overshadowed to rejoice in the tiny miracles of my changing, growing family. That 4th birth was amazing, and my son, Zion, is now grown. He shines in every possible way.

As women loving ourselves and appreciating our own beauty really contributes to our happiness. I like to start and end my day with a little prayer of appreciation for all the blessings in my life, my family, my home, my village, the sun above and the rain that makes our food grow, the air we breathe, my garden, and my healthy beautiful body.

Also try to say this simple blessing to yourself, each time you catch your own image in the mirror: "You are so beautiful, I Love you."

Love is like a nutrient. Try to surround your self with love, for love is that secret ingredient, that makes our food taste better, it helps us digest, and assimilate the vitamins and minerals in the food. The sun, rain, wind, earth, and farmers, pour love into the vegetables that end up on our tables. When we enjoy their bounty with love, the circle of life resonates.

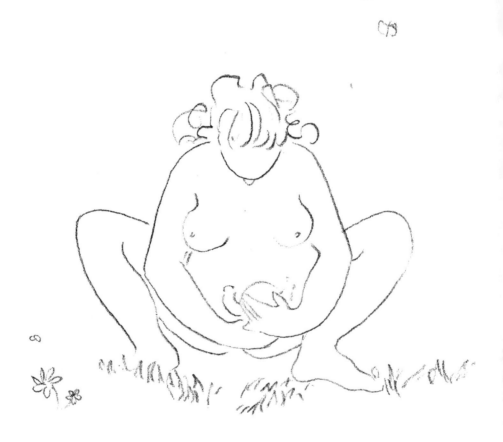

"The wisdom and compassion a woman can intuitively
experience in childbirth can make her a source of healing
and understanding for other women."

~ Stephen Gaskin

The Power of Three...

A Three legged stool stands strong, even on bumpy surfaces. I believe in a three-legged approach to motherhood, respecting Culture, Nature and Science. As a midwife, doula, sister, mother, auntie and grandmother, I find that I am best able to support a woman on her journey, as she navigates through the waters of pregnancy, labor, birth and postpartum, if I humbly bow to these three aspects of healing medicine: **Culture, Nature and Science.**

The Earth is populated by so many beautiful diverse cultures. Culture will determine for a woman what she will be comfortable with. Will she be able to eat certain foods? Will she wish for many family members to support her during labor and childbirth? Or, will she prefer to be more private? Will she wish for quiet in the labor room, or joyful chatter? If a woman knows in her heart that she can say the prayers she feels will guide and strengthen her in labor, all will go more smoothly. If she is made to be ashamed of her culture, or is worried that she will be judged, her birth process could be impaired. It is best for families to help the expectant mother to choose a care provider and a place of birth that helps her feel safe, supported and comfortable. At the Yayasan Bumi Sehat (Healthy Earth Mother Foundation) birth center in Bali, where I have been a midwife spanning two decades, we welcome and help Hindu, Muslim, Christian, Buddhist, Catholic, Jewish, and Animist families. We look after women from many countries. Most of the women we help are not at all prosperous and many are indigent, yet they all feel blessed as they get the same loving service at the Bumi Sehat Birth Center. The Bumi Sehat midwives strive to hold a loving space so no one will feel judged, and everyone feels supported. Receiving respectful care is the #1 most important first step to achieving safe motherhood.

Nature must be respected along the journey to motherhood, after all BIRTH is a natural ancient process that works. Look at how very many humans there are on planet Earth. We have been an enormously successful species. I believe that the success of human beings is based on the fact that we need love to reproduce and love to accomplish the natural process of birth. Making love abundant costs nothing! Love is built into Nature's blueprint.

Oxytocin, released by our pituitary gland, is the hormone of love. It is the essence of the hormone oxytocin, which we feel when we share a meal with friends and family, it is the warmth of singing songs, of holding hands, of gazing into your soul-mate's eyes. In fact, looking into any pair of loving eyes inspires a surge of oxytocin. Love, without a doubt is the most tender, yet powerful force on Earth, for love drives us sexually and it is by way of the miracle of sexual union that we are able to bring children into this world. The love hormone drives sex, and opens the only doorway to this planet. Surely, this is the planet of love, for love alone gets us here.

Arriving on Earth with LOVE, sets the pace for a life lived in love. That primary love spills over to family, friends, community, society, and it sets us up to love and protect our Planet. Love sustains Gaia, our home. Love is our hope, our only hope.

The nature of oxytocin inspires us to make love, to make babies. It causes our uteri to contract in labor and drives the birth machine. Afterward it is oxytocin that prevents dangerous maternal postpartum bleeding, by contracting the uterus so that the birth will be complete, the placenta born, and the bleeding abated. Oxytocin in concert with prolactin, released from our anterior pituitary gland, plus a myriad of hormones and nutrients makes lactation possible. We make our babies, we birth them and we may feed them due to the miraculous nature of the love hormone dancing in harmony, inside of our bodies, with a cocktail of many amazing hormones.

Animals and humans transport hormones via their blood. Plant hormones are carried by sap. Hormones spur cells and tissues to grow and regenerate. This is the secret of how plants sustain our bodies and how they may heal us humans and animals, if we are ailing. So very tiny, in fact microscopic "spirits" which look crystalline, yet hormones regulate our moods and guide our life force, and make the entire dance of life possible. During pregnancy and lactation hormonal activity is greatly enhanced. You can see why we must respect nature when it comes to caring for pregnant women and their babies.

Choosing natural foods, breathing fresh air, and drinking pure water, avoiding all that is unnatural is the key to respecting nature. Protecting the Earth in your choices, for example, buying locally grown foods and products, and planning to breastfeed, are valuable steps in securing this planet's safety, for your baby.

Choosing BirthKeepers (also called a healthcare providers), midwives or doctors, who work with doulas and respect the natural spiral of pregnancy, birth, postpartum, breastfeeding and parenting, will help ensure your safety and that of your baby.

"How could you give a vaginal exam to a mother tiger in labor? What would happen if you took a mama bear's cub away after she births?"

~Sister MorningStar,
Cherokee Midwife and Catholic hermittress

Science is the fascinating academic branch of midwifery care. When we need science, and apply it wisely, it can save lives. For example, I don't feel it is important to know what sex the baby is, I love a mystery. Of course in modern times, we have a choice to find out the sex of our babies before birth, with ultrasound scans. Just remember, our Divine Creator did not put a window on our bellies, so I feel the secret is sacred, and part of the fun, is in not knowing. I ask our back-up Obgyn, to avoid telling couples the sex of their baby when they do an ultrasound scan. In fact, unless there is a situation in which an ultrasound scan is needed, I do not recommend it routinely. If there is a need for a scan I say: "Better living through science." And we do it. At Bumi Sehat we do have an ultrasound scanner, but we use it seldom, and only when indicated. Unless the couple really wants to know the gender of their baby, we do not even look for it.

Sometimes we need the help of obstetrical science to safely navigate the waters of pregnancy and birth. Applied with respect for nature and respect for culture, science can be a very effective blessing. The benefit of any technology must outweigh any potential risks. Technology is best used wisely, only if needed.

"Consciousness.... It turned into the first impulse of intelligence contained in the first cell that became you and me, no more than a flicker of life at the moment of conception and yet containing the total information of the universe."

~ Deepak Chopra M.D.

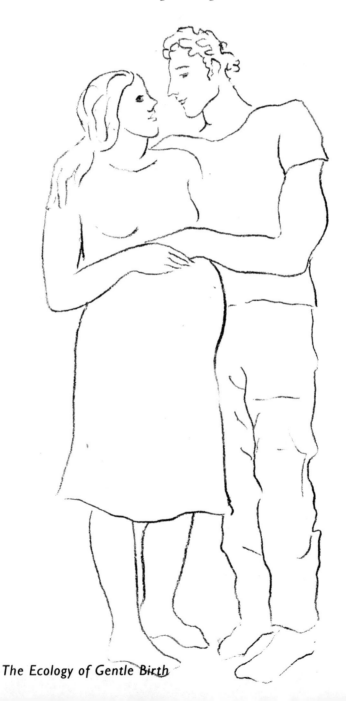

Conscious Conception

As a woman, remembering the warmth of your lover's touch, you may wonder, "Will a child actually be produced from such sharing? It seems unbelievable. So many times we've been close, with no new life springing forth. How can I be sure that a child will grow within my body now? Will my body know what to do? Will I know what to do, what to think, how to feel?"

As you ponder these questions, there is tremendous activity deep in the most private recesses of your body, living activity, which you can visualize. Once it begins, and conception takes place, buckle your seat belt, for the process is miraculous, it unfolds like a living mandala. You cannot control it, but you may support it, by making wise, natural choices, even before conception, if possible.

> *"I am circling around God, around the ancient tower,*
> *and I have been circling for a thousand years.*
> *And I still don't know if I am a falcon,*
> *or a storm, or a great song."*
>
> *~ Rainer Maria Rilke, 1889*

What you do have control over is preparing the garden of your uterus and entire body, for the growth of the baby. You can do this by surrounding yourself with love, drinking plenty of pure water, and eating wholesome nutritious foods. I advise my daughters and all women wishing to conceive a baby, to begin taking an organic, bio-available (meaning our cells really absorb and utilize the nutrients), prenatal vitamin and mineral supplement, even before becoming pregnant.

If you are having relations without family planning, (that's called planning a family) simply begin prenatal vitamin and mineral supplements in anticipation of conception.

Avoid pollution both environmental and emotional. If you walk to work or attend school along a very busy road, with lots of emissions from automobiles, try to plan a new walking route, which avoids the poison. At the gasoline pump, allow someone else to fill your car, so you do not breathe the fumes, also avoid allowing the gas to get on your hands and permeate our skin. Women planning to conceive and those who are already with-child, must not handle gasoline and other menacing chemicals, like toxic cleaning products.

Arguments and stress are emotional pollution, this has adverse affects upon you and your tiny newly conceived baby. I once lived beside neighbors who habitually argued. When they found they were expecting a baby, the arguments became louder, as they were under great stress from many directions. I asked them to consider the baby, when an argument began, and for one of them to simply call time out by saying, "Peace, peace, our Baby can hear us." Within a few days, the arguments stopped, they told me they began to understand that peace was always available between them. Sometimes just calling time-out caused them to cry, and hug, which is a great way to release stress. They had a lovely daughter.

Your baby is developing so fast, by eight to ten weeks of gestation she or he looks like a tiny complete person. Maybe you do not look pregnant yet, but you may be feeling the effects of the pregnancy on your body and spirit. Rejoice… you are already a mother!

If you have made any mistakes, perhaps before you realized you were pregnant, please don't fret. Remember cortisol, the hormone of sadness and stress also has ill effects upon baby. From the moment you suspect you have conceived a person, a baby, make better, healthier choices, to protect this developing human.

Fertility

For many couples achieving pregnancy can take some time, so please don't panic or get discouraged if you do not fall pregnant very quickly after you decide to have a baby.

Men should keep in mind that their sperm count is greatly reduced if they smoke cigarettes. That includes tobacco and other things that are smoked.

For both men and women fertility is improved by following wise nutritional advice. The suggestions in this book are a good place to start.

Men are generally fertile all the time, unless there is an issue like, low sperm count. Women can get pregnant only when they are ovulating, this occurs during our monthly cycle, and our fertile time lasts only a few days.

We know when we are fertile because we women are like the Mother Earth, when it rains, we can plant seeds and they will grow. When a woman's yoni feels wet or moist, she is most likely in her fertile time. If you tune into your body, you will be able to know the difference between wetness from arousal and wetness from fertility. Or wetness from ill health (can be itchy, and smell not-nice), or perhaps wetness from semen (which has a particular smell) and is present after you make love.

Some couples avoid making love when the woman's yoni feels wet because they think the fertile mucous is unclean. This is just the opposite of truth, when a woman is wet she is in her very special time of ovulation and possible fertility. When a woman is fertile, she will likely be more attracted to her partner. When you feel or observe wetness or mucous, especially the slippery kind, like the white of a raw egg, this is the time to let your partner know you are fertile, so that you can make love, and if you are blessed, achieve pregnancy. For more specific instructions on how to determine your symptoms of possible fertility, look for information about the Billings Method of Natural Family Planning.

Note: If the discharge from your yoni has an Unpleasant odor, and/or if your yoni is itchy or painful, and uncomfortable please see your midwife or doctor.

If your moon cycles (menstrual cycles aka your "period") are regular and normal and If you have not achieved pregnancy after six months of sexual relations without using birth control, it would be wise for both the man and the woman to be evaluated by a Doctor of Traditional Chinese Medicine (TCM). If your cycles are too short (21 days or less), or too long (36 days or more, from the first day of one menstrual bleeding to the first day of the next cycle), you should not wait, quickly begin to see a doctor of Traditional Chinese Medicine. Usually within 3 cycles after beginning treatments with a TCM doctor, your cycles will become normal, and pregnancy is more likely. The doctor of TCM should check and treat both the man and woman for possible underlying health concerns that may be preventing conception. Often it is simply that your circulation is stagnant, which impairs fertility in both men and women. Blood stagnation, also called stasis, is often easily remedied by acupuncture, and correctly prescribed herbs. Keep in mind that it may take many treatments to fully resolve fertility issues. It takes time to diminish fertility, and it may take time to replenish it. On the other hand, I have known very fortunate couples whose fertility was restored in just one acupuncture treatment, after years of trying to conceive a baby, because the problem was a simple one!

Other couples have had to seek treatment on a regular basis for many weeks or months. Adjustments in your lifestyle, and wise food choices, may be suggested by your doctor of Traditional Chinese Medicine (TCM). I suggest seeking the help of a doctor of a TCM before seeking more technological solutions to fertility issues, because I have seen the effectiveness of TCM. For example at the Bumi Sehat clinic our doctors of TCM were able to help a couple conceive, who had tried "In Vitro Fertilization" (IVF) twice, without success. Another couple paid dearly for "Intrauterine Insemination" (IUI), they had sold the family rice fields, to pay for the procedures, until they were broke and discouraged. They sought acupuncture, given freely at Bumi Sehat, and were prescribed specific herbs, after nine weeks of treatment they conceived. They had a daughter, and are now expecting a second baby. Modern medical techniques of achieving pregnancy are often successful, the science of IVF is quite amazing, but because they do not treat the underlying health issues, sometimes the mother will miscarry the IVF baby, so dearly wished for.

I always tell women that my goal is not to get them pregnant, my goal is to prepare them to carry a child. When they are balanced and the body is capable of holding and carrying a child, they will achieve pregnancy on their own. Similarly, the beauty of marrying western fertility treatments with TCM is that IVF/ IUI can most certainly help couples conceive – it's now a science – but it's the TCM treatment that actually supports a healthy pregnancy to term.

~ Jennifer Surjana, Doctor of TCM

Of course, if the natural methods, like observing and charting your symptoms of possible fertility also known as, the Billings Method, and TCM don't help you achieve pregnancy within a few cycles, it is time to seek the help of an allopathic fertility specialist. However, you would be wise to still see the Dr of TCM, to optimize your health, before and after conception. To prevent miscarriage, continue to see the Doctor of TCM throughout your pregnancy.

The Bumi Sehat midwives have helped several couples that conceived by IVF and IUI methods. These couples sought the most natural midwife-to-mother prenatal care and childbirth option, in addition to continuing to have acupuncture treatments throughout pregnancy and postpartum. Just because one has achieved pregnancy with the help of science, does not mean an automatic cesarean birth.

When you decide it's time to have a baby begin preparing your body right away. You can do this by taking good quality organic prenatal vitamins. Also, vitamin E 400 units a day has been found to improve fertility in both men and women. Coq10 has been found to boost the quality of the mother's eggs, in therapeutic doses of between 100 to 600 mg/day.

I can't say it enough times: No smoking. Drink plenty of pure water. It has been shown that making love regularly, a couple of times per week, increases sperm supply. If you make love very infrequently, sperm supply decreases, so make LOVE. Practice makes perfect!

Vegetarian Mom's-to-be, you MUST ingest protein. Soy is no longer a good choice of vegetarian protein, as nearly all of it is GMO and tainted with glyphosate, a dangerous killer.

Midwife and fertility researcher Jacquelyn Aurora advises vegetarian people seeking to conceive, to consider: Getting essential B Vitamins, necessary for conception and growing a healthy baby, from a low mercury fish, and organic eggs 1 to 2 times per week at least. Super foods, like Royal Jelly, Maca found in South America, Goji, found in Asia, can be good sources of nutrients that support fertility and nurturing of life in your womb. There is an excellent book: The Vegan Mom-to-Be by Wendy Louise Hagler. Wendy gives excellent advice on how much protein a mom-to-be needs daily, and how to get it via beans, nuts and other plant based foods. If you are already in your mid 30s and are ready to conceive, don't wait too long to adjust your lifestyle in readiness for pregnancy, birth and parenting.

> "My husband and I tried for eight years to have a second baby. The first one was easy to conceive, but that was before we were vegan. We were so discouraged. Our midwife advised us to eat some high quality meat protein. It was hard for me to let-go of being a complete vegetarian. We decided it was really important to welcome at least one more child into our family, so we did eat some very good wild caught fish, and we began to take yogurt and some tasty organic cheese and eggs. Like magic, within my next menstrual cycle, I was pregnant!"
>
> ~ Tina, now the mother of three

How "FATHER" Nature Chooses the Gender of Your Baby

All women's eggs may become either a male or a female child. The sex of the baby is actually determined by the individual sperm of the father. Men who smoke should know that cigarette smoking kills a significant percent of his sperm and the male sperm are more vulnerable. Smoking greatly reducing the chances of having a boy baby.[1] Also smokers should know that smoking tobacco damages sperm DNA.[2]

Male sperms, called Androsperm, have long tails and smaller heads. They are stronger and swim very fast yet they live only a maximum of 24 hours. Female sperm, called Gynosperm, has short tails and fat heads, they swim slowly and may live up to 5 days in the fertile environment of the cervical crypts and uterus of an ovulating woman. Wet mucus is life supporting.

When women have just begun to ovulate, and there is just a bit of wetness evident at the entrance or just inside of her yoni, if she makes love, she will most likely conceive a girl. While the boy sperms reach the egg first every time, if you have sexual relations in the early days of fertility, the egg is not yet ripe, the boy sperm die waiting to get inside. Meanwhile the girl sperms have taken their time arriving at the egg just when it ripens and softens to allow one sperm to enter. Thus, a girl is usually conceived under these circumstances.

If the ovulation process is well on its way, and the woman waits to make love until she has slippery mucus or slippery wetness, that has a stretchy character, like egg white, she will more likely conceive a boy, if she and her partner make love that night or day. This is because the mother's egg is ripe and ready when the faster swimming boy sperms reach it first, one of them goes right in. The girl sperm arrive too late. It's all in the timing.[3]

You can think of the race for the egg, like the story of the Tortoise and the Hare. The female sperms are Turtles, slow and sure, strong, wise and long-living. The male sperms are like quick running rabbits, athletic, lightning fast, and always first to arrive. But first is not always the winner. This is how Mother Nature and Father Time work in concert, so we may have both male and female babies.

NOTE: If you very much need to have a baby boy, perhaps for cultural reasons, do not make love at all, until the slippery fertile mucus is evident at the vulva of the woman, this increases your chances of having a male baby. IF you have already made love, during the days/nights of early wetness of fertility, before you feel slippery, and then make love again when the slippery mucus is evident, your chances of having a boy are still only 50-50.

If you wish to conceive a daughter, make love only at the very onset of fertile symptoms, when wetness first appears on the first day or two of possible fertility, then stop, wait and see what happens.

Pregnancy

Healthy Tips... While YOU Are Pregnant....

- Drink plenty of pure water.

- Eat green vegetables everyday... Organically grown if possible.

- Eat fresh fruit as often as possible... Remember to eat a rainbow of colors.

- Eat protein every morning and evening. like eggs, fish, chicken, organic meats, nuts, seeds in combination with whole grains, organic dairy products like: cheese - not the soft cheeses, yogurt, milk if your body tolerates it.

- Include healthy fats in your diet: butter & cheeses from grass fed cows, olive & coconut oil.

- Eat 3 or 4 or more meals a day, 2 is not enough!

- Take an organic prenatal vitamin & mineral supplement, that includes folate (not folic acid), everyday.

- Avoid foods and spices that contain MSG, also called Vitsin, this flavor enhancer is a poison.

- Choose wholesome natural staple foods, like red or brown rice, quinoa, barley, millet, oatmeal, hearty dark whole wheat bread.

- Cut back on eating sweets, craving sweet foods means your body needs protein. Sugar interferes with the insulin balance in your body and inhibits how your assimilate fat. Don't diet, if you are worried about your weight, cut back on sweets.

- Foods like yogurt, kefir and naturally made sauerkraut, contain probiotic and are very healthy for your digestion. Bonus: Healthy digestion helps to inspire healthy mental health.

- Take a nice walk every morning and evening.

- Think happy thoughts … it helps make your baby smarter, really!
- Sing to the baby in your belly, baby hears you and loves it! This is an important job for your partner, baby can hear the voice more clearly, that can get closer to baby-belly.
- See your midwife for regular prenatal check-ups, so she can help reassure you and help you stay healthy.
- Conception to 28 weeks: Monthly prenatal check-ups
- 29 to 35 weeks: Check-up every two weeks
- > 35 weeks gestation: Weekly check-ups, or more often if indicated
- Choose a midwife and/or a doctor who you trust, who cares about you, believes in you, and who shares your vision for what your birth can be, should everything unfold in a natural healthy way…
- Plan to have your birth in a clean place nearby your home, (or at home) which has a very low rate of cesarean births.
- Hold this in your heart … that most women can birth in a normal healthy way. BELIEVE

"Touch is the first language we speak."

~ Stephen Gaskin

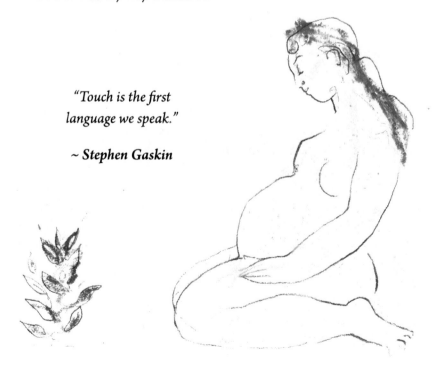

May We Make Love During Pregnancy?

If there has been NO spotting or bleeding, no unusual cramping, and you have no history of miscarriage, you and your partner may enjoy making love gently. Remember, the prostaglandin in semen is absorbed into the pregnant mother's blood stream, and we know that this amazing hormone increases health and intelligence for the baby, especially in the second trimester, when fetal brain development is most profound.

If you have had some spotting, cramping or threat of miscarriage, abstain from intercourse until after the 20th week of pregnancy, or until your healthcare provider has given you the green light. The prostaglandin in semen does soften the cervix and orgasm can cause mild practice contractions toning your uterus, so IF there is NO threat of miscarriage, making love can get one ready for a nice labor.

Choose positions that are comfortable. You will need to be more creative as your belly grows bigger. Remember, you and your partner must be faithful so that there is no risk of endangering your baby with a sexually transmitted infection.

If you have some spotting after making love, it is usually because your cervix is more fragile than normal. However, it's a good idea to see your midwife or Obgyn about it.

Dreams...

Quite often pregnant women have very vivid dreams. This increase in dreaming may be due to those amazing pregnancy hormones. It may also happen because the growing baby moving in the womb wakes the mother, so she can remember her dreams. It may also be due to the fact that pregnancy is a heightened state of spirituality. Usually the dreams are peaceful and joyful, but sometimes they can be disturbing. All of these kinds of dreams are quite normal please do not be alarmed. Scary dreams are usually a way for us to release stress. Nearly 40 years ago, when I was a young woman expecting my first baby, I would dream that the baby was flying away in the night, and coming home at dawn. It frightened me, but I grew accustomed to my little time traveler doing her thing.

My first baby dream was about a baby girl. Later I dreamed of a boy... and I had a girl. I have noticed that with each of my pregnancies, the first dream I had of the sex of the baby, was correct. I would also dream of asking the baby to help me choose her or his name. This was repeated when my second grandchild was gestating, I dreamed his parents were walking with him, calling him "Bo." When he ran too far ahead of them they called out, "Bodhi... Bodhi." The next morning my daughter-in-love took one look at me and said, "You had a dream about our baby, I know it! I tried to refrain from telling them my dream, for I wished for my son and his wife to choose their own baby's name. Well, the mother-to-be persisted, and when I finally told her, she was very pleased, and Bodhi Padma Edzra Banjo Bernhardt, had his name. Many pregnant women, and their families, dream that they are learning how to understand the baby's true heart and soul, I call this kind of dream a "Wisdom Dream".

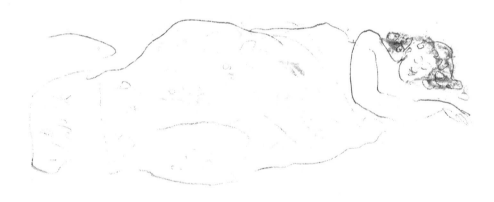

"We can do no great things...
only small things with great love."

~ Mother Teresa,
recipient of the 1979 Nobel Peace Prize

Things to Avoid During Pregnancy....

For the health and well being of your baby, and for yourself, absolutely avoid alcoholic beverages.

You must not smoke or take illegal drugs, and you should avoid being near other people when they smoke or take drugs. Regarding all artificial substances, like MSG, artificial sweeteners, and food additives, when in doubt, leave it out. If you are on any medications, be sure to tell your doctor, or nurse practitioner, that you are pregnant, right away, and every time you see them. Even better; if you are planning to become pregnant, talk to your doctor and your midwife, about any prescription and or non-prescription medicines that you may be taking.

Regarding caffeine, like coffee, strong black tea, instant coffee, soft drinks, chocolate and cocoa drinks, these should only be taken in moderation. Avoid all artificial sweeteners.

Some companies advertise the sale of milk products especially for pregnant women. However, many people have difficulty digesting dairy products. If milk products do not agree with your tummy, don't drink them. If milk and products containing milk do agree with your digestion, then you may wish to enjoy them. Some cows are fed RGBH, you must be careful not to drink the milk of cows fed this dangerous growth hormone. Meat and dairy products, these are concentrated foods therefore it is quite important to choose organic. Your baby will not suffer if you cannot drink milk while you are pregnant, for there are many ways to get plenty of calcium. Leafy green vegetables, especially if you squeeze a bit of lemon on them, contain calcium. Some people who cannot digest milk can enjoy yogurt, another source of calcium, with no problem.

Avoid: meats that are raw or under cooked, like sushi, packaged meats, like 'hot dogs', soft cheeses (sorry no Brie cheese). Also cut back on fried foods. Laxatives should not be taken.

Environmental pollutants like air pollution or toxic waste, are a hazard for your baby. Avoid busy streets where the air quality is bad, and dump sites that may contain all kinds of dangerous waste. Chemicals used in farming, gasoline, kerosene, strong cleaning solutions, all should NOT be handled by pregnant and breastfeeding mothers. If your work involves handling this kind of chemical, speak to your employer about it, and ask that your duties be redefined, to protect your baby.

Burning of plastic garbage in not only bad for our environment, it is dangerous for us to breathe the smoke. Please stay away from all burning garbage.

Cat and bird feces sometimes contain Toxoplasma gondii parasites, a harmful organism, which can cause damaging infection, called toxoplasmosis, to be passed to the baby. Expectant mothers should never handle animal droppings. Someone else must clean the cat litter box. Also, you should wear gloves while gardening, to avoid contact with cat feces in the soil. After enjoying touching your pets, always wash your hands thoroughly with warm water and soap. Also to avoid toxoplasmosis infection, never eat raw or under cooked meats. If you already have made antibodies to toxoplasma gondii, before you get pregnant, your baby is protected.

Places with lots of strong electrical cables and cell phone towers create electromagnetic fields, which may harm your baby and increase the risk of miscarriage. Also, avoid x-rays, if you must have an x-ray ask your doctor for extra protective covering. Please, do not sleep with your cell phone, or computer pad.

Please Do Not Fast...

Fasting is a controversial subject, as a pregnant woman you are feeling more spiritual, and therefore if you are Muslim, you may really want to join in the Ramadan fasting. It is however not required and it is best if you do not fast while you are pregnant and breastfeeding. If I may show you the Muslim text regarding fasting: Hadith as narrated by Anas bin Malik, says that the Messenger of Allah said: "Certainly, Allah excused the traveler of fasting and a portion of the salah, Allah has also excused the pregnant woman and the breastfeeding woman of fasting" (Tirmidhi).

A devote Muslim mother may fulfill her obligation by feeding a poor person, rather than fasting while pregnant and breastfeeding. This solution protects her baby, while upholding her fine level of feeling for her religion.

Fasting in very early pregnancy may put the baby at risk for birth defects. Throughout pregnancy it increases the risk of miscarriage and small-for-dates babies, also known as, intrauterine growth restricted babies, who may have a more difficult time surviving after birth. I am quite certain that our Divine Creator considers each baby precious, and wants the mothers to do all they can to protect the next generation, including eating and drinking wisely and plenty, while pregnant and breastfeeding.

Sometimes mothers-to-be have eating disorders. This is a kind of illness, and should not be judged, however, it must be dealt with immediately. If you are greatly limiting your food intake, or dieting, or choosing only a few kinds of food, or only one kind of food, or causing yourself to vomit after you eat, you must share this with your health caregiver, right away. (Vomiting from pregnancy nausea is different than causing yourself to vomit habitually.) If you look in the mirror, and see a body that is big and revolting, rather than a body that is blossoming with life, you should be concerned about having an eating disorder. Another symptom is feeling that because of your restricted diet, you are above, or better than, other people. One mother told me that her "food guru" believes it is ok to fast on water while pregnant. I found this "food guru" on line, and indeed he does advise fasting on water, while pregnant. I wish I could take this misguided advice off of the web. It's just not right for the mother and it is unfair and dangerous for the baby, to fast on water only while pregnant. Please don't do this, and avoid all fad diets.

There is strong correlation between epigenetic changes caused by starvation often due to war, forced migration, strife, and fad dieting (low calorie, low carbohydrate, limited diets) during pregnancy, that may predispose the gestating children to obesity in later life.[4, 5] Because our planet is changing and to be honest, 'times are hard,' an expectant mother may feel she is losing control, and the one thing she may feel she has control of is her weight gain. This may have a profound ill effect upon her body image and the gestating baby's wellbeing. If you find yourself responding to the stress of modern times and pressures by greatly limiting your food selection and intake, seek professional help right away. Please, mother-to-be, don't starve for two.

All mothers-to-be worry; "Will my baby be all right?" The best we can do in pregnancy and as new mothers is to avoid potentially dangerous situations, think positive thoughts and offer up our fears to the Divine Creator. Please try not to worry too much, as excessive worrying can also be harmful to you and your baby.

Coping with the Discomforts of Pregnancy

"I am the decedent of many strong women who all gave birth successfully. Every cell of my body knows how to be pregnant and how to birth my baby."
~ Deborah Flowers

Nausea

Though they call it 'morning sickness' many pregnant women experience nausea all day. If your nutrition is poor the nausea will be more acute. This means avoid 'junk' foods like snacks made with white sugar and white flour. Also avoid deep fried foods. Instant noodle soups that contain MSG, are not a healthy food choice.

Severe nausea…. If you are vomiting nearly all the food and drink that you are taking, you may be getting dangerously dehydrated. This is called hyperemesis gravidarum. You will need to see your health care giver plus follow the nutrition guidelines in this book, to make every bite of food count. You will need to push yourself to eat and drink. Acupuncture, Homeopathy, Cranial Sacral and/or Chiropractic therapies are often very effective in turning severe pregnancy nausea around. Your biggest challenge will be to stay well hydrated.

Nausea Busters

- Eat many small meals throughout the day and a protein snack at night.
- Drink mild ginger root tea.
- Eat baked or steamed sweet potato with salt (to taste).
- Take high protein snacks, like hard-boiled egg, strips of organic chicken, yogurt, nuts.
- Enjoy fresh fruit and or try rujak (see recipe in this book).

Heartburn

Later in pregnancy, the baby's size pushes up on your belly, while your hormones cause the muscle separating your esophagus and your stomach to relax a lot. This causes heartburn. It will be cured once you have had your baby. In the meantime try these tricks....

Heartburn Busters

- Avoid all spicy foods – NO sambal, hot salsa or Hot Spicy Sauces!
- Drink young coconut water and eat the soft coconut meat too.
- Take an after meal walk so your food may digest, avoid laying down too soon after eating.
- Sip warm milk or take a tablespoon of fresh cream, when you feel the burning.
- Avoid drinking and eating at the same time, it slows down digestion.
- Keep raw nuts like cashew or almonds in your pocket, eat often, chew well.
- Eat papaya, fresh and or dried, often. It will help your digestion.
- Eat baked sweet potato or white potato with just a bit of salt or gomasio.
- Avoid alcohol beverages and caffeine – they stimulate excess stomach acid.
- Eat smaller meals, for frequently.

Constipation

Many pregnant women suffer from constipation. Pregnancy hormones, which help prevent miscarriage also keep the wind in your body moving upward, instead of downward, this can make it more difficult to pass stool. Remember, you must drink plenty of fluids, like pure water, fruit and vegetable juices, healthy non-caffinated teas. Eating plenty of wholesome foods, like fresh fruit, salads, lightly steamed vegetables, and whole grains, will help as they contain roughage and prevent constipation. Junk food on the other hand can cause constipation. Constipation commonly goes hand-in-hand with headaches. This may be due to a build up of toxins in your body, hormones, stress, a stiff neck or dehydration.

Constipation Busters

- NO Laxatives while Pregnant!
- Drink plenty of fluids; water, fruit and vegetable juices, healthy teas.
- Eat roughage, found in fresh fruit, salads, vegetables, whole grains.
- Dry fruits, soaked in water, currants, raisins, apricots, figs and prunes really help.
- Avoid junk foods, made with white flour and white sugar, they stop you up.
- Stay active, go for walks, do yoga or go swimming, it will help promote regular bowel movements.
- Take a good quality probiotic supplement

Hemorrhoids

This aliment is sometimes caused by constipation. Take the steps above to prevent painful hemorrhoids. Sometimes it runs in families, perhaps due to the family sharing the same dietary habits. I had five term babies, and never got a hemorrhoid. I was among the fortunate, perhaps due to good eating habits I learned from my Filipino mother, lots of fruits and vegetables. My husband (Who obviously has never been pregnant, nor has he given birth!) has suffered most of his life from hemorrhoids. Everyone in his family also suffers. They grew up on a very American diet of white bread, meat and junk food. Pregnancy certainly can cause hemorrhoids, or make them worse, due to increased vascular pressure and increased blood supply, plus nutritional strain. Let's face it, it's not a happy situation.

Increase your intake of fresh vegetables, nuts, seeds, beans sprouts, whole grains, wheat germ and fruit. The additional vitamin A, B, C and E will help you heal. Try eating yogurt with fruit, seeds, nuts and wheat germ sprinkled on top.

Nothing helps relieve constipation and abate hemorrhoids better than drinking plenty of pure water.

Taking a good quality probiotic supplement is very helpful as well.

To reduce swelling and inflammation of hemorrhoids try Witch Hazel or ginger compresses, made with fresh grated raw ginger, apply directly. Keep the area clean by washing often with warm water and mild, natural soap, and pat dry. Never use bleaching soaps or strongly perfumed soaps on your body. Gently push the hemorrhoids back inside, apply Hemorrhoid Oil as described below. I have seen this recipe help with even the terrible swollen red, painful kind of hemorrhoids.

Do NOT rush your bowel movements, don't push. Squatting on the toilet, rather than sitting, helps to maintain better pelvic health, however comfort is key.

Hemorrhoid Curing Oil:

3 oz. Castor Oil (choose the odor free, organic)

7 to 11 drops pure Tea Tree Oil

7 to 11 drops pure Lavender Essential Oil

Decant all above oils into a small bottle or jar.

Apply to clean dry area, gently pushing hemorrhoids back inside.

The pressure of the growing baby on your pelvic floor and additional blood volume associated with pregnancy exacerbates hemorrhoids. Most women who avoid constipation and generally keep good health spontaneously loose the hemorrhoids soon after the baby is born.

Aching Back

Back rubs are my favorite remedy. People often ask a pregnant woman, "What can I do to help?" How about offering the expectant mother a massage?

Dancing Hula, belly dancing, pelvic rocks, prenatal yoga, swimming, nice walks and making love all help.

Good nutrition really helps, make sure you are getting enough minerals, especially calcium, magnesium and vitamin C. Take natural prenatal vitamins. Try to choose an organic prenatal vitamin and mineral supplement. I personally had an aversion to taking pills each time I was pregnant. I was happy to find an organic prenatal supplement that combined and balanced calcium, magnesium, additional vitamin C, plus it contains probiotics and herbs to support pregnancy. My favorite vitamin and mineral supplement for expectant mothers is "Perfect Prenatal" made my new Chapter in Vermont. This made it possible for me to get the nutrients I needed, in one pill. It did help alleviate my nausea and backache.

If your back is aching, please tell your midwife, so she can check you for kidney tenderness. During pregnancy a mother-to-be's kidneys can come under great stress. Your midwife or doctor will check you to be sue your backache is not due to unhealthy kidneys. Doctors of Traditional Chinese Medicine are quite skilled at alleviating kidney stress. Gentle Cranial Sacral Therapy and Chiropractic care are quite effective in alleviating many discomforts of pregnancy.

Itching and Skin Conditions

Most itchy skin in pregnancy is caused by stretching and hormonal changes. Gentle, massages with oil (almond, sesame, coconut, olive, avocado, apricot or vitamin E oil) help a lot, as do warm baths with flower petals and a few drops of pure flower oil, try rosemary or lavender. Some essential oil companies have brilliant blends for MotherBaby.

Make sure your clothing, towels and sheets are washed in mild laundry soap and well rinsed. Pregnancy can make you more sensitive to irritants like detergent residue in your clothing. Choose cotton or natural fiber clothing over polyester or blends.

For a few women itching skin during pregnancy can really get intense. This is often due to the body's efforts to purify, releasing old stored toxins through the skin. Detoxification causes excess heat in the liver and blood, which must be released via the skin, this is why it itches. It can feel like you are on fire. This is known as a condition called PUP (puerperal uticaria). Try drinking the water of young coconuts and eat the soft flesh. Coconut is an ancient remedy, to relieve the excess heat in your body. Cut fried and fatty foods out of your diet. Drink more water. Eating steamed or raw beetroot has been found to help. Sometimes with PUP nothing seems to help except finally having the baby. Even if you are really uncomfortable PUP does not harm mother or baby, you must try not to scratch so much that your skin become raw and sore.

Anti Itch Salad:

- 1 Beetroot ~ peeled and grated
- 1-2 tbsp lemon or lime juice
- 1-2 Tbsp Omega oil (best) or Virgin Olive or Coconut Oil
- Natural Soy sauce ~ to taste
- Toss together and enjoy!

Melasma or 'mask of pregnancy', is characterized by discoloration of the skin, mostly on the forehead, nose and upper lip. Melasma is not usually itchy, but it makes women feel very self-conscious. Caused by hormonal changes, it gets worse if the mother is nutritionally stressed and it gets darker if exposed to the sun. Covering your skin to protect it from the sun helps minimize this condition. It normally goes away gradually after the baby is born. Improved nutrition is the key. In some Native American tribes, mothers would rub the baby's first poo, the meconium, on melasma to reduce the staining of the skin. I have not tried this, but it can do no harm.

Itchy vagina especially if accompanied by strong odor may be a vaginal infection. Try sitting in a warm sitz bath with a few tablespoons of apple cider vinegar, for at least 20 minutes, three times a day. If after three days the symptoms persist, please tell your health care giver. Avoid making love until it clears up completely. As pregnancy comes to its fullness it is very important to clear up any vaginal infections so the baby won't be infected as he or she passes through the birth canal. Wear cotton underwear only, or none at all, especially at night while you sleep. Wipe after bowel movements only from front to back, to prevent infecting the vagina with feces. Wash with mild soap (or no soap) and water at least twice daily. Never douche, unless your health care giver recommends it.

Pregnancy does increase the wet and juicy quality of your vagina. There will be more discharge. If your vaginal discharge has no unpleasant odor (like bad fish or too-yeasty) there is no infection. You simply are more-juicy, a condition naturally occurring in pregnancy. Increased heat due to additional body weight, increased blood flow and hormonal levels contribute to a vaginal environment that has a more delicate balance and needs protection against infections.

For the same reasons mentioned above, you may also sweat more, while pregnant and breastfeeding. This is just your body's natural ecology,learn to love it.

Swelling

At the first sign of swelling of fingers, hands, feet, ankles, or face, drink more pure water. Swelling is a message from your body saying: "Take better care of me!" You may be sweating a lot and not getting enough salt. Try Gomazio (see recipe in this book). Or, you may be over salting your food. Salt to taste, but taste your salt. Often mothers-to-be who experience swelling are protein deficient. Are you getting at least two small servings of protein everyday? Swelling means you must pay more attention to getting more nutritious food. Instant noodle soup is not a wholesome meal. If you are eating instant noodles a lot, you are not properly nourished.

Swelling by itself is not dangerous, but you must see your midwife as soon as possible, and have your blood pressure checked to rule out any danger to your self or the baby. If you notice swelling and/or headaches and/or blurry vision, it is absolutely necessary for you to immediately get a check up. Your blood pressure should and must me monitored.

Severe headaches of sudden onset after the sixth month of pregnancy can signal toxemia, a dangerous condition. Your midwife or doctor will determine if your blood pressure is high and if you are at risk for toxemia or preeclampsia.

To reduce high blood pressure:

- Drink more pure water
- Watermelon – eat a lot of it.
- Cucumber – eat one or more whole peeled cucumber everyday
- Onion – eat raw
- Garlic – try plain raw or dice two cloves garlic mix with 1 tablespoon honey
- Prenatal vitamins – a good quality supplement, taken daily or as directed
- Vitamin C with bioflavonoids – up to 2,000 mg daily
- Fresh ocean fish – do not fry try it, best to fire-roast, bake or make soup.
- NOTE: Farmed Salmon is inflammatory and can make the problem worst.
- Stress reduction – prayer/meditation/Reiki/massage/soft music… let go of worries
- Gentle exercise – walking, swimming, prenatal yoga, dancing…
- Choose anti-inflammatory foods: almonds, walnuts, ginger, turmeric, sweet potatoes, beets, dark leafy greens, bell peppers, berries, extra virgin olive oil, etc.
- Avoid inflammatory foods: refined carbohydrates like pasta and white rice, white sugar, white flour, junk food, all cause inflammation which may lead to hypertension.

Miscarriage

About 20% of all pregnancies end in miscarriage, many so early that the mother may not be sure yet she is pregnant. Other miscarriages may occur much later. All pregnancy losses are potentially traumatic and heartbreaking. Usually by 20 weeks along in the pregnancy the risk of miscarriage is very low.

If you are experiencing cramping, and/or bleeding, or low backache, this is called a 'threatened miscarriage'. All hope is not lost, there are some things you can do to prevent the miscarriage, but only if your baby is healthy. If there is something not exactly well with the placenta or the baby, nature will most likely take it's course, and the miscarriage will proceed, no matter what precautions you take.

Other causes of miscarriage are, hormonal imbalances, loose cervix, infections, nutritional deficiencies, maternal exhaustion, or exposure to too much pollution. Often the mother does not ever know what or IF any particular factor caused her miscarriage. Accepting is difficult, especially when one cannot find an explanation. I wish I could offer some comfort, but miscarriage just hurts.

Preventing a miscarriage is possible in some instances. Spotting (passing a scant amount of blood) alone does not mean you have lost the baby. Panic and stress increase the risk of miscarriage, so it is necessary to stay calm and treat yourself with love and care.

If you are spotting, inform your midwife about the occurrence. Complete bed rest is the first step to miscarriage prevention, get up only if you need to use the bathroom. Ask your family and or friends to help you. They can bring you meals, good books and magazines, set you up to view movies at home, etc.

While pregnant you must never lift anything heavier than a newborn baby, especially if you have had some signs of threatened miscarriage. A new baby is usually about 3 kilos, so that is the limit for a healthy pregnant woman to lift. If you have had signs of miscarriage lift nothing, go to bed, contact your midwife and/or doctor, follow her instructions.

Abstain from all sexual activities if you experience signs of threatened miscarriage. Do not resume love-making until all signs of miscarriage have been gone for three to four weeks.

Avoid all cold-natured foods if you have signs of miscarriage. Iced beverages, anything right from the refrigerator, even fruit juices and salads, are "cold" and must be deleted from your diet until the threat has passed plus three weeks. The womb must be a warm place to sustain pregnancy, so it makes sense to choose warming foods. Some warming foods include, miso soup, chicken soup, porridge, sweet potatoes and all root vegetables like carrots, beets, and white potatoes, leafy green vegetables. Sip warm water, rather than cold fluids.

Prenatal vitamins, choose wisely, making sure they are truly natural. Vitamin E and vitamin C in reasonable doses, can reduce the risks of miscarriage. Do not take large doses of vitamin C. Make sure you are getting enough protein, like, hard boiled organic eggs, fresh small ocean fish, natural chicken or beef. Vegetarian mothers-to-be must take special care to get enough protein and nutrients.

Doctors of Traditional Chinese medicine have acupuncture techniques and herbal formulas to "hold the baby". You may be wise to consult one. Your regular doctor or midwife may recommend a skilled Doctor of Chinese medicine. I have seen acupuncture and carefully prescribed Chinese herbs save very wanted pregnancies, which were at risk. These babies are growing up healthy and strong. Mothers who have experienced miscarriages in the past, and are again expecting, should see a Doctor of Traditional Chinese Medicine as a preventative and to maintain optimal health, and prevent chronic miscarriage.

Not every miscarriage can be stopped. If the cramping continues and the bleeding gets worse and/or if you pass clots and tissue, pregnancy loss may be inevitable. Nature may just take her course and your body may be strong enough to complete the miscarriage on its own. In this case, letting the miscarriage happen naturally and spontaneously is the more gentle way. However, you will want to see your OBGYN doctor to determine if the miscarriage is complete. Incomplete miscarriage carries the risk of hemorrhage and/or infection and can affect your future fertility. A complete miscarriage can be confirmed by ultrasound. Incomplete miscarriage may require a D&C

(dilation and curettage of the lining of the uterus) or acupuncture to facilitate the passing of all articles of conception. Until all the bits that have died have passed out of your uterus, it is difficult to process the emotional and spiritual trauma of miscarriage.

While suffering from a miscarriage you will want to rest, keep warm, allow a loved one to rub your feet and lower back, drink plenty of warm water. Avoid all sexual intercourse, as your cervix is open and vulnerable to infections. Welcome the help of people who care and love you. They can help you cope with the disappointment and sadness. A hot water bottle on your belly can help you cope with the cramping.

If your pregnancy is far enough along you may pass a recognizable tiny baby, or even a bigger baby. Try to make a ceremony, to bury the tiny Baby's body. Planting flowers or a tree, including a love note in the little burial site, are all good ways for the broken heart of a mother to mend.

Warning: Women experiencing miscarriage should not be left alone. ... There is grave risk of hemorrhage. If you feel clammy, spaced-out, anxious, incoherent, or pale, someone must take you to the hospital immediately as these are symptoms of shock, and you are in grave danger. After miscarriage, if there is foul smelling discharge, or your temperature becomes elevated, you must seek immediate medical help.

If, in spite of your prayers and efforts to hold the pregnancy, you still loose the baby, try to know in your heart that YOU have not failed. Grief, disappointment, even guilt are normal emotions after such a loss. The midwives at Bumi Sehat Bali, where I normally work, have looked after many women who have lost one or even more babies to miscarriage. Later, many of these same, sad and brokenhearted mothers, had healthy happy babies.

We encourage women to begin a program of good nutrition, prenatal vitamins and healthy lifestyle, even before they fall pregnant again. Allow yourself to heal from the trauma of the pregnancy loss, look for help if you are not coping well. Sometimes some good cries with your partner, midwife or a close sister or friend, can help release the stress and set the stage for a healthy pregnancy to unfold in the future. Sometimes miscarriage mothers need more help and more time to heal. Your body will need to cope with hormone changes, which can make your emotions more acute. Try to be patient with your healing and grieving process, it takes time to let go. The point is not to forget the lost baby, but to heal. I believe the angels celebrate even more than usual when a mother who has suffered pregnancy loss, has a healthy full term baby. Some mothers may never carry a baby to full term, and they are to be loved and respected also as mothers. Their miracles may not be growing up in our world, but they are indeed, miracles.

Some people try to rush you to "Get over it." They may even say, "It was only a miscarriage, at least it was not a baby!" You did have a Baby! Your Baby. Do not listen to people who try to minimize your loss, they may be just coping with their own suppressed feelings of loss. When you allow yourself to cry and release in a healthy grieving process, you will heal faster and more completely. Healing cannot be rushed, but when it is supported, it flows more smoothly, and Mothers who have lost children, may once again open to life.

My son Zion shared something astonishing when he was fourteen years of age. He told me that he could remember his siblings, twins, a boy and a girl, who died before birth, and who played with him and stayed with him, while he was deciding to be born. I had indeed miscarried twins, a boy and a girl, at 22 weeks gestation, ten years before Zion was born. They were just about the size of my hand, and perfectly beautiful. I had never mentioned the twins to my living children, though I had often wondered what becomes of the souls of miscarried babies. Zion's story confirmed my feelings, that when we lose tiny babies, even as miscarriages, they remain a part of our family. Perhaps some babies come back, and are conceived and carried by the mother. Others find a place elsewhere, in the great mystery. After hearing Zion's story, my other children agreed, they also knew their unborn siblings. They had played together in a place my children call heaven!

Premature Birth

If you go into labor before 37 weeks gestation, it is considered premature. I support mothers to birth with midwives if they have completed 36 weeks of pregnancy by dates. Some midwives must adhere to more strict regional rules. Generally 36 weeks gestation is the cut off for a homebirth.

Remember, you may have remembered the date of your last menstruation incorrectly. If you had an ultra sound scan early in pregnancy, the date of predicted delivery is more accurate than dates obtained later in pregnancy. Some women have shorter or longer cycles, which would mean their "due date" may not be "average." So it's best not to panic. Many mothers who thought they were having babies at 35 weeks, turned out to be much more along than they imagined. The field of Obstetrical Medicine is now reconsidering the issue of gestational age.

If you feel cramps that have a definite beginning and end, and or see some blood or brown discharge, you may be going into labor too soon. Do not panic. One common cause of premature labor is maternal exhaustion and stress. Call your midwife or doctor. While you are waiting to be checked, you must rest 100%. If it is determined, that you are indeed in labor, you will have some decisions to make. If your amniotic waters have released, your baby will be born soon. You will be closely monitored to avoid risks of infection.

Your doctor or midwife will measure your belly, and/or use ultra sound to determine your baby's approximate weight. If your baby is over 2.5 kilos and fetal heart rate establishes that baby is handling the labor well, labor will most likely allowed to proceed naturally. Remember that babies born vaginally have fewer breathing problems than babies born by cesarean birth.[6] Premature births are normally best handled in the hospital, where special care can be easily accessed, if your baby needs it.

I have received many babies into the world who at 36 weeks gestation were perfectly ripe and big enough to need no medical care at all. They did need immediate and constant skin-to-skin contact with mother and exclusive breastfeeding.

If your baby is indeed premature a good way to stop labor is to see a Doctor of Traditional Chinese medicine. They have acupuncture methods and herbs to "hold the baby."

If baby does come early or is term but of a low birth weight, Kangaroo Care is best. This means that instead of an incubator to keep baby warm, the baby should be swaddled between your breasts, skin-to-skin. Mother's body perfectly regulates and provides the exact warmth the baby needs. The baby should be fed breastmilk exclusively. If he or she is too weak to suck, then you may pump your breasts and feed the baby your colostrum by tube, cup or spoon until he or she gains weight and strength. This will take resolve, as many hospitals prefer to keep premature babies in incubators and feed them with IV fluids. More and more hospitals are considering the Kangaroo Care research, and supporting it as optimal care for premature babies.

The best way to prevent premature labor is throughout pregnancy; eat healthy wholesome foods, avoiding MSG, get plenty of rest. Avoid pollution and drink plenty of water and other healthy fluids. Do not lift anything heavier than a newborn baby while you are pregnant. That means no more than 3 kilos (6.6 lbs). Avoid too much exposure to the hot sun or saunas, and make sure you stay well hydrated. Avoid all medications, unless prescribed by your doctor or midwife and make sure he or she knows you are pregnant, before you take any medications. Reducing stress is very helpful in preventing miscarriage, I know, easier said than done. If in spite of your efforts, you birth your baby early, please don't feel guilty. If your baby requires hospitalization, you may have a bumpy road ahead, and will need your energy for healing your baby, not feeling guilty. Some early babies require only skin-to-skin with Mother and Father, and exclusive breastfeeding.

One Mother shares her premie story...

"My Baby girl Rose, came at 32 weeks, minus 2 days. I was under tremendous stress with the father of my baby. I did not take adequate rest, nor did I eat and drink properly. I was moving away from my partner, so I was lifting boxes of my belongings, against the advice of my midwife. When my water released, I was devastated. I felt that my dream of natural childbirth was shattered, along with my dream of the perfect family.

I was so worried about my baby. Our midwife took us to the hospital, where I was bedridden, on IV fluids, we tried to hold the baby, medically and with acupuncture. We hoped to buy some time so my baby's lungs could mature. Four days later, contractions began. Our midwife had been coming regularly to hospital, bringing healthy foods, and support. Our ob-gyn doctor and our midwife were a good team, friends, colleagues, who shared a vision for gentle birth. The hospital administration tired to get us to sign a document waiving skin-to-skin, accepting that baby go strait to an incubator for observation, and allowing them to clamp and cut our baby's umbilical cord immediately. Our doctor and midwife assured us that this document did not represent the best of evidenced based care for a premature baby, or any baby. So we refused. A bully hospital administrator tried to then force us to leave, but I was pushing, so our doctor kicked him out of the room. Five hours after my first contraction, while my doctor and midwife sang Gayatri Mantra, our favorite spiritual song, I was on my hands and knees and my daughter was gently born. There were no complications at all for me or for baby. She arrived with her eyes wide open, 1 kilo and 900 grams (4.188 lbs). She gave a lusty cry and went right to my breast, to suckle. Our hearts broke open. We stayed one more day in hospital then transferred to our midwife's home, to help make sure our baby was breastfeeding well, gaining weight and thriving.

I kept my newborn Rose, skin-to-skin, continuously for the next eight weeks, because I wished for her to have the opportunity to continue gestating and growing, if not inside my womb, at least very close and touching me. I ate and slept and listened to soft music, skin-to-skin with my baby. When I went to the bathroom, I would give her to my partner or a close friend, to hold, also skin-to-skin, until I quickly returned.

My partner and I are not getting married, but I am ok with his commitment to co-parent with me. As a 38 year old first time mOm, I feel blessed that our daughter, Rose, chose me. I love being a mOm, and her father loves being a dad."

~ Kimberly, a mOm who survived premature birth, with her perfectly healthy baby

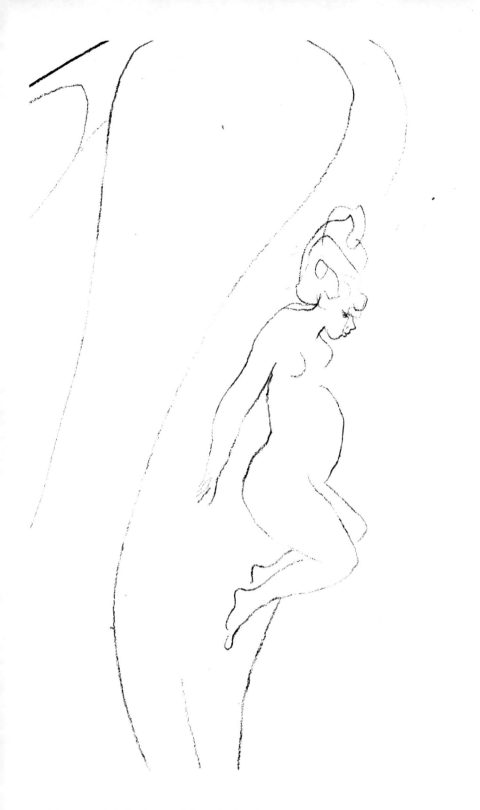

Eating For Two

Remember that you are eating for two now... in fact, if you are carrying twins, you are eating for three! This does not mean you must eat twice as much, though you will need to increase your calorie intake by 1,000 calories per day while pregnant, and 1,500 calories per day while breastfeeding. It does mean you must be twice as conscious of eating healthy natural, organic foods to nourish your body, so your baby will be healthy.

Fortunately most human cultures support expectant mothers in eating well. If you wonder what you should be eating, ask your grandmother, or your great grandmother. Her generation ate mostly natural wholesome organic foods. They did not simply eat quick junk foods from the package, full of MSG, artificial colors and sweeteners. They had fewer modern conveniences like junk foods. Our grandmothers most likely had kitchen gardens and ate healthy organic vegetables and fruit on a daily basis. In climates with cold winters, our grandmothers would grow vegetables and fruit, and preserve them at home, in glass jars. One could still see the fresh healthy colors of the tomatoes and cherries in the jars nestled in Grandma's basement! Sauerkraut was something many of our grandmothers made and served. Now many nutrition experts are saying that old-fashioned sauerkraut is full of healthy enzymes and probiotic organisms therefore very good for us.

Again we can talk about the 'Power of Three' we have a culture of eating well, there is of course the natural healthy way, and then there is the science of nutrition to guide us to eat properly as mothers.

Importance of Protein

Every cell of your baby's developing body is built with protein. We need wood to build a house. To build a body for your baby, the house of his or her soul, you need to eat protein, for protein is like the wood, the structure of the house. A small amount of protein, twice a day is essential for maintaining optimal health during pregnancy.

The list below includes both vegetarian and non-vegetarian sources of protein. Vegetarians should be sure to combine legumes and with whole grains and nuts to get complete proteins.

Sources of Protein

- Eggs – choose organic eggs from free range chicken.
- Tofu and Tempe– make sure you have a clean organic source, not made with formalin. Look for non-GMO and organic.
- Soybeans, steamed fresh, green (edamame).
- Black, pinto, red beans, etc... beans are best if served with sesame, peanuts, red or brown rice for complete protein.
- Garbanzo beans
- Cheese – avoid soft cheeses in pregnancy
- Yogurt – choose a healthy unsweetened natural yogurt, or make your own at home
- Peanut butter, almond butter, cashew butter, sesame tahini
- Sunflower or pumpkin seeds
- Raw nuts
- Meat ... beef, chicken, turkey, fresh water or sea fish. Small deepwater fish are the best source of protein and Omega oils, which promote brain development in baby. Large fish may be high in mercury, and should be eaten only occasionally. Meat, eggs and dairy are very concentrated foods, therefore it is doubly important that you make sure your feed your family only organic. The extra cost is still a bargain, when you consider the value of your family's health.

Fat is Essential

So much popular belief in what constitutes a healthy diet is based upon fads that equate a skinny body with health. Being very overweight is of course a strain on all systems of the body, and should be avoided. However, somehow FATS got a bad rap. The human brain needs fat to function optimally. I am not saying go ahead and eat a kilo of fatty pork per day, not a all. I am saying that all people, especially people who are expecting babies, must ingest some healthy fats, everyday.

Healthy sources of FAT:

- Grass Fed Butter
- Ghee (clarified butter)
- Virgin Olive Oil
- Coconut Oil
- Fish oil ie Omega oils, found in small ocean fish, you may also take it in capsules
- Organic meats
- Walnuts, pecans, almonds, macadamia nuts, Brazil nuts, cashews

Iron Rich Foods

The best protection against anemia and hemorrhage following childbirth, is to load up on iron rich foods, during pregnancy. Prevention is indeed the best medicine.

If you eat iron-rich foods along with foods that provide plenty of vitamin C, your body can better absorb the iron. Try a squeeze of lemon or lime on your steamed leafy greens.

Remember, dark leafy greens Prevent anemia, they are great sources of iron and calcium

- Egg yolks
- Dark, leafy greens (spinach, collards, kale, tatsoi, broccoli, chard, sweet potato leaves, water spinach, water cress, etc.)
- Dried fruit (prunes, raisins, apricots, peaches)
- Iron-enriched whole meal cereals and grains
- Mollusks (oysters, clams, scallops)
- Turkey or chicken giblets (choose organic)
- Beans, lentils, chick peas and soybeans
- Liver
- Artichokes
- Red meat
- Pesto made with fresh Basil (also contains olive oil, a source of healthy anti-inflammatory fat)

Simple Vegetables ~ back to basics

Vegetables should be organically grown and eaten fresh. You may eat vegetables raw in salads, or just crunch into a crispy red or yellow bell pepper. When cooking vegetables I prefer to steam them quite lightly, so keep the color and vitamins. Sometimes a warm bowl of freshly steamed broccoli, with melting butter is just the perfect snack. Add Sesame Gomazio over brown or red rice, and you have a nutritious meal. When choosing vegetables, eat the colors of the rainbow, because each has something healthy to offer you.

Planting a small vegetable garden, even if it is just for leafy green vegetables and salad is a wonderful investment for a family. Home-grown food is more nutritious, as it is picked fresh, prepared and eaten, before the nutrients are lost. I try to always have basil growing in my garden, so I can make Pesto in a heartbeat. Gardening is very good for your body and soul. Please remember not to use chemical fertilizers or pesticides on your little garden, for they are dangerous.

Growing food organically is so important for our health today and for future generations. Fresh picked leafy green vegetables from the garden or the market provide us with so many important minerals, like iron to prevent anemia. Paku fern, and any leafy greens are easy to make. Just rinse the leaves and toss them in a hot wok with a dash of sesame oil and organic soy sauce or liquid aminos or sea salt. You may wish to add a squeeze of citrus and bit of grated ginger and/or turmeric, to make your food even healthier.

"How could we have ever believed that it was a good idea to grow our food with poisons?"

~ Jane Goodall, Harvest for Hope: A Guide to Mindful Eating

The Importance of Red & Brown Rice... healthy carbohydrates

Midwives and doctors are wondering, "Have women forgotten how to give birth?" This is a very good question when you look at the rising rate of cesarean birth. You would think that modern women are healthier than their grandmothers were, but it may not be so.

The introduction of "Green Revolution", white rice, also called "Miracle Rice" or "High Yield Rice" in the late 1960s and early 1970 changed the staple food of most of Asia and the rice-consuming world. Our grandmothers and great-grandmothers enjoyed eating red rice or brown rice that was a whole grain, this rice provided them with complete nutrition.[7] Wholesome grains are healthy carbohydrates, which pregnant women need to grow the baby within. Other healthy carbohydrates include: quinoa, millet, whole grain porridge, oats, organic sweet potatoes, (any organic tubers are good), black rice, pasta made with whole grains.

In Indonesia, it has been found that one of the leading causes of death is hemorrhage after childbirth.[8] These deaths are caused by maternal malnutrition.

I believe they are preventable. If one speaks with the Dukun Bayi, the Traditional Midwives who attended women at birth before there were hospitals, they will tell you; that the problem of women bleeding at such an alarming rate after childbirth, is a modern one, it began to happen more often soon after the rice was changed, from nutritious red to high yield, fast growing white rice.

For this reason I ask women to serve their family organic red rice or organic brown rice or other wholesome grains. It makes a huge difference in how you feel and definitely improves your nutrition with many benefits for you and your baby. I know the red rice or brown rice, is more expensive, but your health and the health of your family is precious. Invest in good wholesome foods today, to prevent serious illnesses later in life. Even though the price of red or brown rice per kilo is higher than the price of white rice, one gets so much more nutrition from eating wholesome red or brown rice varieties.

Research has also proven that eating red rice porridge after childbirth will bring the mother's milk in faster and the volume of milk will be more.

Folate vs Folic Acid

Folate is the naturally-occurring form of vitamin B9, important even before conception, to prevent neural tube defects in the baby. Folic acid is the synthetic form of the vitamin, very different from the natural form. Folic acid is found in most prenatal vitamin supplements and in fortified foods, like "enriched cereals" There is now a growing awareness that while Folate is essential, Folic Acid may be having some harmful effects. Just to be sure, be sure to choose a vitamin supplement that has Folate in it, NOT Folic Acid. Foods rich in Folate rich foods include: peanuts, garbanzo beans, navy beans, pinto beans, lentils, spilt peas, black-eyed peas, corn, spinach, asparagus and, beef liver. Best to begin eating these Folate rich foods, before you even achieve pregnancy.

Some Nutritious Recipes for the Childbearing Family

"Life is always a rich and steady time when you are
waiting for something to happen or to hatch."

– E.B. White, Charlotte's Web

Pesto

This recipe is suitable for people who prefer to eat only raw foods, simply do not toast the nuts and the garlic. It is a fantastic vegan source of protein (from the nuts), iron, vitamin A & C, and healthy fat (olive oil). Pesto is a good pick-me-up. When you feel low on energy, eat a couple of tablespoons of pesto, right from the jar. Keep it refrigerated. You may eat it on toast or crackers, toss it with healthy pasta, mix it with brown or red rice, and eat it with salad.

Ingredients:

- 4 to 6 ounces (100-200 grams) fresh organically grown Basil leaves (Ocimum basilicum) Note: I mix sweet basil with *kemangi* (Indonesian or Thai basil) and *tulsi* (holy basil), depending upon what is growing in my garden.
- 1 cup (or about ¼ kilo) of raw cashews (or toasted in a dry pan until golden)
- 2 to 6 cloves Garlic ~ optional (peeled, raw or lightly toasted)
- juice of ½ medium to large Lemon or 2 Limes
- 1 cup extra-virgin organic Olive Oil
- Salt to taste

Fill blender with freshly picked organic basil leaves, add the lemon or lime juice, olive oil and begin to blend on medium speed. Add the garlic, and cashews, a little at a time. Blend or pulse, adding salt to satisfaction, until all is well ground into a coarse green paste. Enjoy the fresh rich flavor.

Red Rice Milk

This very nutritious beverage is easy to make from ingredients that are easy to find in Indonesia. In Mexico it is called Horchata. Research has shown that red rice and red rice milk, if taken postpartum, increase mother's milk supply. If you add the cashews the milk will be richer and creamier in texture, plus the nuts add protein.

I often add a banana to the last step in the blender, as a treat for the children. This is a good addition to any vegetarian diet. People who are allergic to dairy may enjoy this lovely animal free "milk".

Ingredients for concentrate:
- 200 grams organic red rice, rinsed
- 1 liter pure water
- 1 cinnamon stick
- 50 grams raw cashew nuts (optional)
- ½ vanilla bean (optional)

In a large saucepan, combine rice, water, cinnamon stick, vanilla bean and cashews. Set aside to soak for minimum of 3 hours. I like to soak it overnight. After soaking, bring above ingredients to a boil, reduce heat, and simmer for 40 minutes to 1 hour. Allow to cool.

Remove cinnamon stick, puree cooked and cooled rice mixture in a blender until smooth. Strain through a fine sieve. Set aside as your concentrate.

In the blender combine:
- 225 ml rice concentrate (above recipe)
- 250 ml pure water
- 25 ml palm sugar or raw honey to taste
- pinch of sea salt

Blend until smooth. You may make it thicker or thinner as you desire by adjusting the amount of water. Rice milk may be served warm or cool. Makes a very nice milk for tea or chai, or a base for fruit smoothies. Try flavoring it with ground cardamom spice, mango, banana or almond extract, experiment to find your family favorites!

Golden Almond Milk

This milk is the perfect postpartum warming drink for mother. It will help to balance the wind in her body, which is quite all over the place after childbirth. Soothing, healing and a help in bringing in mother's milk. Whenever a new mother breastfeeds her baby, some should bring her a cup of something wonderful to drink. This will be a favorite.

Ingredients:

- 1 cup blanched almonds
- 1 ½ cup pure water (for soaking, later discard this water)
- another 1 ½ cup of pure water
- 1 inch of fresh turmeric root peeled and diced (or ½ tsp. of powdered turmeric)
- 1 to 3 large soft pitted dates
- pinch of salt

Place almonds and water in a bowl, cover and refrigerate for 4 to 6 hours or overnight. Drain away water.

Put soaked almonds and a new 1½ cup of pure water in the blender with a peeled 1 inch piece of fresh diced turmeric root, 1 to 3 large pitted dates, and a pinch of natural sea salt. Blend on high for 2 to 3 minutes, until it is smooth and creamy.

Strain through cheesecloth or a medium-fine kitchen strainer. Serve warm to make it more soothing.

Sesame Gomazio

All people, especially pregnant mothers, need salt in balance, too little or too much is dangerous and can aggravate hypertension, and edema (swelling of hands feet and face). A good way to make sure you are getting enough salt, but not too much is to make up this recipe for Gomazio. Remember that in the Middle East the sesame is called "The Seed of Immortality". Sesame is rich is calcium, protein, vitamins A and E, zinc, copper, magnesium, phosphorus, iron and potassium. Always choose real sea salt, as it contains iodine, to prevent goiter. You may use gomazio to flavor all your foods, instead of plain salt.

Ingredients:

- 1 cup raw or roasted sesame seeds. (White sesame seeds are cooling, which means they are best for people who have a lot of heat in the body, like growing children and people of hot temper. Black sesame seeds are warming and have more benefit for people with cold in their bodies, like older people or those easily chilled).
- 1 ½ tsp sea salt
- 2 tbsp spirulina and/or moringa oleifera (optional)

Roast sesame in dry skillet on low heat stirring continuously so the seeds pop but don't burn. Just as the seeds become golden brown add the salt. When slightly cool, grind all ingredients in a, dry mill, blender or traditional mortar and pestle, until coarsely ground, not too powdered.

Try sprinkling it generously on everything, a hardboiled egg will become a gourmet snack with gomazio on it. It adds protein and calcium to salad too. Add to any food, for a calcium rich flavor, with not-too-much salt. Sesame added to whole grains makes it a complete protein, easier for the body to assimilate.

Moringa Oleifera leaves or dried powder (called Malungay in Philippines and Daun Kelor in Bali) dry the leaves and add to Gomazio. Moringa leaves, dried or fresh, or powdered may be added fresh to porridge or smoothies. They are a source of iron as well as a galactogoue, known to increase breastmilk!

Chicken Adobo

This is a specialty of the Philippine Islands, in fact this recipe is from my grandmother, who was a Hilot or Dukun Bayi (traditional healer and midwife). She would tell me that Chicken Adobo could cure any illness. When someone in the family would get *masuk angin* (wind in the body), my "Lola" would make her famous Chicken Adobo. Her recipe has more vinegar than most, which may be why it is so healing and balancing. Choose organic, free range chicken.

Ingredients:

- 1 kilo chicken – cut into 4 to 6 cm. parts
- 4 to 6 cloves garlic – crushed and peeled
- 4 to 6 black peppercorns
- 2 bay leaves
- 6 white potatoes – cut into 3 - 4 cm cubes
- 2 carrots – cut into 2 to 3 cm pieces
- ½ cup apple cider vinegar
- ⅓ cup soy sauce
- 4 cups hot water
- pinch of brown or palm sugar

Heat a large deep stainless steel pan. Toss in the chicken parts with the garlic and bay leaves. Stir the chicken and garlic while searing at medium to high heat in the pan, until it is just a bit golden brown, 7 to 10 minutes. If you have left the skin of the chicken on, it will have it's own oil for braising. If you have removed the skin, you should add a couple of tbsp olive oil. Add the vinegar, soy sauce, sugar, potatoes, carrots, and peppercorns, cover. Simmer for 10 to 15 minutes. The potatoes will now be about half cooked. Now add the hot water.

Reduce heat to medium-low and allow the Adobo to cook for another 30 minutes or more. The longer you simmer the Adobo, the more tender everything becomes and the flavors meld. Serve with hot steamed red or brown rice.

Hawaiian Shitake Tempe

Tempe is quite easy to find all over Indonesia and now in the USA, and it is an economic source of protein. Try to find organic GMO free Tempe. Sweet potatoes are like medicine for the uterus. Leafy greens like spinach, are a great source of iron to build strong blood cells. Shitake mushrooms are an anti-oxidant to move toxins out of our bodies.

Ingredients:

- 6 to 8 Shitake mushrooms fresh or dried (if dried soak for half an hour in water or until tender) – cut into thin strips
- 1 block Tempe – cut into 2 to 3 cm cubes
- ¼ cup olive oil
- 3 to 4 cm piece fresh ginger – sliced very thinly
- 1 small green papaya – open, remove seeds, peel and cut into 2 to 3 cm cubes
- 2 medium sweet potatoes, wash and cut into 2 to 3 cm cubes
- 2 medium carrots, sliced into 2 cm rounds
- ½ kilo green beans or long beans – cut into diagonal bite sized pieces
- ¼ kilo leafy greens of your choice
- ½ cup soy sauce
- ½ cup inexpensive wine (Red or White) or beer.
- ½ cup drinking water (if you soaked shitakes, use the soaking water)
- Black or white pepper - to taste

Soak dried shitake mushrooms in warm water until soft, cut into thin strips. Fresh shitake: simply wash and cut into strips, set aside. In a large stainless steel pot or wok brown Tempe with oil and ginger, for about 10 minutes, stirring frequently so it does not stick.

Add soy sauce, water, wine or beer, sweet potatoes, papaya, and carrots. Cover and simmer over medium heat for about 10 - 15 minutes, or until carrots and sweet potatoes are nearly cooked through. Add green beans and mushrooms and lastly leafy greens. Allow to simmer a while longer, only until tender, do not over cook. Remember vegetables that still have their color and are not mushy, still have their vitamins and minerals. Serve with brown or red rice and gomazio.

Gado-gado

A traditional Indonesian medley of fresh healthy vegetables flavored with peanut sauce, a good source of protein. Tofu contains calcium and protein, sweet potatoes are nourishing for the female reproductive system. A perfect food, for pregnant and breastfeeding mothers and their families. Any or all of the vegetables listed below may be used or try your own combination. Choosing local vegetables in season is healthier for your body and for our planet.

Ingredients:

- ¼ kilo green beans
- 1 broccoli stalk
- 1 small head of califlower
- 2 sweet potatoes
- 2 potatoes
- 1 to 2 carrots
- ¼ kilo mung bean sprouts – washed, bean hulls removed
- ¼ kilo water spinach
- ¼ kilo spinach or kale
- 1 kilo firm tofu

Gado-gado Sauce:

- ½ kilo raw peanuts
- 4 cloves garlic
- 2 cm piece of Laos root grated (or ½ tsp dried Laos) or small piece of fresh ginger
- 2 small chili peppers
- 50 grams palm sugar (or brown sugar may be used)
- 2 – 3 tbsp soy sauce
- 1 tbsp olive or coconut oil
- pure water as needed to thin sauce

Cut all the vegetables you wish to use into bite sized pieces, steam until tender, about 5 minutes. The root vegetables will take longer, so put them in the steamer first, adding the leafy green and tofu last. Set aside while you make the sauce.

Saute peanuts on a dry skillet, stir constantly so they do not burn. Dice all of the spices and chili peppers and fry together in olive or coconut oil until fragrant. Combine ALL ingredients with red sugar and soy sauce in blender or use traditional mortar and pestle, add water to get consistency you like, thick but still able to pour.

Arrange steamed vegetables and tofu on serving tray serve sauce on the side or pour it right over. Gado-gado may be served by itself as a snack or a light meal.

Rujak Sehat

A favorite recipe from our Asian great-grandmothers, rujak is very nutritious, full of vitamins and it helps relieve pregnancy nausea.

Sauce: Diramas… kneed together with pure water:

- Tamarind paste – aka *Lunak* (seeds and bits of shell removed/strained out)
- Palm sugar – aka gula Bali (also Mexican brown sugar, or use your local natural sugar)
- Small chili peppers, use the mild kind, aka *Cabe rawit kecil* – dice very gently small
- Salt to taste

Peel and cut into bite sized pieces any of the following fruits or vegetables to be dipped in the sauce:

- Green mango
- Jicama aka *bankuang* or *singkamas*
- Apple and/or pear
- Ripe pineapple
- Sweet orange or tangerine peel and divide into sections
- Cucumber –peeled and sliced thinly

Rujak is best enjoyed with friends and family, sitting around the kitchen table, dipping and talking and eating.

Miso Soup

Miso is a protein rich paste of aged soybeans. It is easily found, often in the Japanese food section of the super market. This recipe is easy and quick to prepare. It is warming to the body, nourishing with iron, and it tastes lovely.

Ingredients:

- 2 sweet potatoes – cut into 2 to 3 cm cubes
- 4 shitake mushrooms – if dried, soak 1/2 hour in warm water and slice thinly, use this mushroom water for soup later.
- ¼ kilo soft tofu – cut into cubes
- ¼ kilo leafy green vegetable of your choice (try watercress)
- 3 or more red onions (shallots) – diced
- 1 to 2 cloves of garlic – peeled, diced
- 1 to 2 inches of ginger root peeled and grated
- Add any rehydrated seaweed you like (optional, wonderful for healthy hair & nails)
- ½ liter of drinking water
- 3 to 4 tbsp miso paste (depending upon how salty you prefer your soup)

Boil all ingredients (except miso) in ½ liter of water, until tender, not mushy. Add leafy greens last, as they cook faster.

Dip out about ½ cup of the soup broth and using a fork stir the miso paste into this cup until it is fully dissolved. Take soup off of fire and add this miso and broth mix last. Serve and enjoy topped with Gomazio.

Pumpkin Soup

Pumpkin meat is diuretic, slightly laxative, calming and strengthens the immune system, perfect for pregnant and postpartum mothers. It is effective when illnesses of the stomach and intestines are present and also in cases of heart and kidney ailments. Traditionally pumpkin was seen a health-restoring aid for people suffering from typhoid fever and dysentery. The healing properties are attributed to the plant's high potassium and magnesium content, which restores the body's mineral balance. Pumpkin and other squashes are a great dietary aid, since ¼ lb of cooked flesh account for a mere six calories.

Pumpkin seeds contain high concentrations of beta carotene, vitamin E and phytosterenes, plant hormones. They promote excellent bladder function, easing cramps and strengthening the bladder muscles.

Ingredients:

- 1 kilo of pumpkin meat – peeled and cut into pieces, steamed until soft
- 2 tablespoons olive oil to sauté spices
- 3 cloves of garlic diced
- 2 inches of fresh ginger root – peeled diced
- ½ large onion – diced
- 1 cup young coconut cream (can be found canned, or made fresh, or you may rehydrate the dried coconut milk)
- Salt to taste
- 4 tbsp roasted pumpkin seeds – for garnish
- dash of ground black pepper

Steam pumpkin meat, mash. In a soup pot warm olive oil, add garlic, onions and ginger, sauté until all tender and aromatic. Add mashed pumpkin and coconut milk, stir well. Keep on medium flame, add pure water to get consistency you prefer for this soup. I stir it with a large wire whisk. Salt to taste. After serving into bowls, top each with a teaspoon or more of the roasted pumpkin seeds or Gomazio and add a dash of pepper.

Black Rice Pudding

This traditional nutritious breakfast or dessert is an Indonesian favorite. Versions of it are found in Thailand, Vietnam, and Philippines too.

Ingredients:

- 150 grams black rice
- 100 grams glutinous rice
- 2 small *pandan* screw pine leaves (optional, available in Asian stores)
- 1 inch ginger root – peeled and crushed
- ¼ tsp salt
- 1 liter water (or more as needed)
- 1 400 to 500 ml tin/box of Coconut cream (or make homemade by grating mature coconut, and mashing by hand in water, strain)
- Fresh fruits (optional) cubed, add as topping.

In a heavy lidded pot, combine black rice and glutinous rice, rinse 3 times and then soak overnight. In the morning, change the water. Add ample water for cooking, add the salt, pandan leaves and ginger root. Bring to a boil. Lower heat and simmer until rice is well cooked. Stir occasionally to be sure the water is enough.

Sauce:

- 250 grams palm sugar (or raw brown sugar)
- 300 ml water
- ½ tsp vanilla extract or 1 inch of vanilla bean

Grate palm sugar (no need to grate if you are using brown sugar) and combine with water in a sauce pan. Bring to a boil and reduce heat to low, simmer until the mixture becomes syrup. Add vanilla, stir. What you do not use for black rice dish may be used to naturally sweeten other things like pancakes.

In the morning serve Black rice pudding warm topped with syrup and drizzled with coconut cream. In the afternoons it is a nice cold dish, served with coconut cream and freshly sliced mangoes, papaya, bananas, strawberries, passion fruit, star fruit, etc.

Mango Salad

This recipe is a natural source of vitamins, calcium and minerals, even protein, plus it's so colorful. It makes a perfect side dish for any meal.

Ingredients:

- 2 ripe mangoes – cut into small cubes
- ½ sweet red onion – diced very small
- ½ red bell pepper – sliced into thin strips
- 2 cups of Lettuce leaves of your choice, torn into bite-sized pieces
- 1 lime – juice of
- A handful of fresh cilantro - diced
- 1 cup raw nuts of your choice (almonds, walnut halves, pine nuts, cashews, etc.)
- salt to taste

Toss all ingredients together and enjoy.

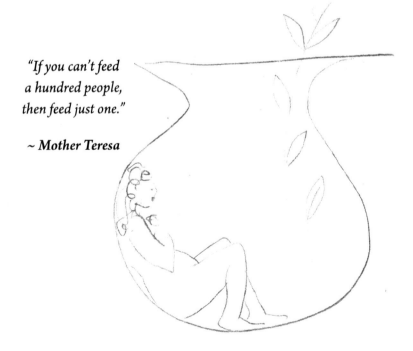

"If you can't feed a hundred people, then feed just one."

~ Mother Teresa

Have a Date

According to the Journal of obstetrics and Gynecology, research concludes that eating 6 dates per day in the last month of pregnancy has many benefits, including: significantly reduced need for induction and augmentation in labor. This fruit of the date palm, a native tree of North Africa, is full of vitamins, minerals amino acids, healthy carbohydrates, fiber, and they taste so good, while preventing anemia. Mothers enjoying dates arrived at the hospitals in labor with more cervical dilation than the mothers who did not eat dates. 83% had good strong amnion and chorion membranes, that stayed intact longer. 96% of the date eating mothers went into spontaneous labor, with no induction, and they were less likely to have pitocin in labor (pitocin enhanced labors are much more painful). Also in the group of date eating mothers, the first stage of labor was almost 7 hours shorter, than non-date consuming moms. (That sounds great to me!) Another study showed that date eating mothers had less postpartum blood loss.

My daughter, Lakota ate dates in her last trimester. She also had regular prenatal care (not prenatal scare). Lakota took organic prenatal vitamins, did regular gentle prenatal yoga and was so excited to be having her first baby. She had a 4 ½ hour labor! My granddaughter, Rimba was born a few days early, a wonderful birth, with no complications.

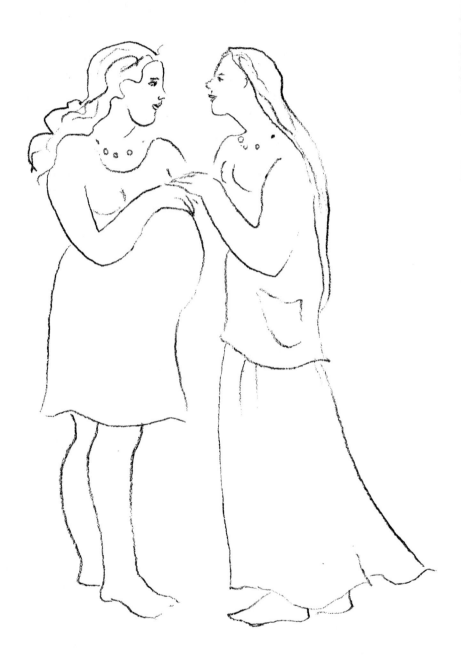

Prenatal Care

Prenatal Care ~ is not meant to be "Prenatal Scare!"

You have a human right to choose who your healthcare provider will be during your pregnancy. Choose wisely, because having a midwife, or a doctor, are very different. Midwives take more time during prenatal care, to really get to know you and your baby. They assess carefully, skillfully and intuitively for risks. Obgyns are skilled at surgical birth. They are a blessing when cesarean birth is really needed. All too often, surgeons feel more comfortable with cesarean, than with natural childbirth. The fact is, if you have a midwife, your chances of having a cesarean birth are significantly lower.

An example; a particular hospital in Bali had 389 babies last year, 367 were born by cesarean, 22 vaginally. The Obgyns at this particular hospital explained that all the cesarean births they did, were medically indicated and necessary. They actually were quite proud of having so many vaginal deliveries in 2015. Bumi Sehat also received 389 babies in 2015, all naturally, gently and respectfully via the Mothers' vaginas. So you see, choosing your healthcare provider is an important decision.

Prenatal care is very important beginning very early in the pregnancy and continuing on through to the birth. After your baby's birth you should have some loving postnatal care. Usually, midwives give more comprehensive prenatal and postnatal care than doctors. At the beginning your midwife and/or doctor will wish to check you once a month. As your pregnancy progresses, at about the 26th week or so, your prenatal visits will be scheduled about two weeks apart. After the 35th week of pregnancy, until birth, your check ups will be weekly. If you have special risks, you will be asked to attend check-ups even more often.

If everything is progressing normally you may just see your midwife. She will give you healthy advice for maintaining your wellbeing and helping the baby grow inside. If she finds risk factors she will advise you to be checked by a doctor of obstetrics. Ask her to help you find one who will likely agree with your childbirth philosophy, and one who works hand-in-hand, heart-to-heart, with your midwives.

Prenatal CARE is not meant to be Prenatal SCARE! If you really have a particular risk, it's best to take your midwife or doctor's advice and work together to find solutions. IF you feel your midwife or doctor is too focused on frightening you, undermining your confidence in your ability to give birth, it's time to consider seeing another healthcare provider, for another opinion.

However, if your midwife and Obgyn agree that your pregnancy has particular risks that make it necessary for you to have your baby in the hospital and perhaps via cesarean birth, you must accept. Sometimes we must employ the science of modern medicine to help us. Wisely employed medical skills do save lives, when they are needed.

Asking Questions… your right and responsibility:

- When is my estimated due date?
- Is my placenta in a good position?
- Is my baby in a good position?
- Do I have plenty of amniotic fluid?
- What is my blood pressure?
- What is my baby's heart rate? (*normal is between 120 and 160 beats per minute*)

These are a few examples of good questions, and you really have the right to know the answers. I am always sad when a pregnant woman does not even know her probable date of delivery. When I ask why the answer is most often, "Well my doctor (or midwife) is too busy and never told me anything. I am too shy to ask." All too often the doctor will do an ultra sound scan and tell the mother the sex of her baby, even if she prefers to keep this a secret. It is as if the sex of one's baby has become more important that vital information to protect MotherBaby's health.

Please don't be shy. It is your doctor or midwife's job to support your health in pregnancy, and to give you vital information. Only with accurate information and open communication do you become "partners in health". Being partners is a wonderful way to help you to stay healthy. So ask questions, share your ideas and dreams and plans. If anything is less than optimal in your check-up, ask how you can correct it. For example, if your blood pressure is climbing up slowly, it is best if you know this and take natural measures to keep it from climbing too high (see the 'Pregnancy' section for tips to maintain healthy blood pressure).

Try to choose health caregivers who resonate with you and appreciate your questions. Remember, YOU ARE YOUR OWN BEST DOCTOR. Your inner knowing will innately give you the most valuable medical advice. The most important healing gift your doctor and midwives can give you is so simple, they must BELIEVE in YOU.

Good sitting positions for getting baby into optimal birth position

Avoid crossing your legs. Sit up straight! Remember, big comfy couches that curve your back and bring your knees up higher than your hips, when you sit, can make the baby go into a posterior position (not optimal, causes longer labors, sometimes leads to transport for instrumental or cesarean birth). If you are relaxing on a couch like that, lay down, take it easy, don't sit crunched up.

When sitting, remember everyday to imagine that you have a golden cord, pulling through your spine, going up through the top of your head, helping your posture stay long and strong. This helps Baby find the best position.

Sitting on a well-inflated birthing ball, with your knees slightly lower than your pelvis helps to bring your Baby into a perfect position for birth.

If when you begin labor, your baby is posterior, choose to labor in the hands-and-knees position, this usually helps baby gently wiggle into a more optimal position for birth. Many midwives know how to Rebozo your belly/Baby to coax Baby into a better birth position. Studying "Spinning Babies" is a good way to help your baby find the best position for both of you, before labor begins.

Mothers, talk to your baby, say… "Tuck your little chin, hands on your heart, look at Mommy's spine. I Love you."

Prenatal Exercise

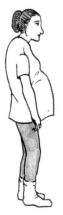

Posture

Proper posture can prevent many pregnancy discomforts.

1. Stand with feet slightly apart, head held high.
2. Shoulders are held back, but not stiffly
3. Lower back does not curve, but remains relatively straight
4. Tailbone is tucked under so your hips do not pull forward

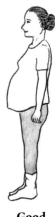

Poor posture

Good posture

Standing Twist

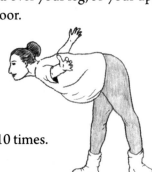

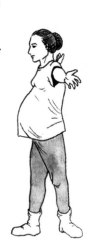

1. Stand upright with feet 12 inches apart. Extend your arms out to each side

2. Exhaling, beind forward at the waist, your upper body parallel to the floor.

3. Inhale to resume the standing position, legs still apart and arms extended. Gently twist to the right, pivoting your right foot slightly.

4. Exhale, bending forward over your leg, so your upper body is parallel to the floor.

5. Inhale and resume the standing position.

6. Repeat, twisting to the opposite side

7. Repeat steps 1-6 up to 10 times.

Squat

1. Stand upright, feet 12 inches apart, knees slightly bent. Raise your arms over your head, with hands joined and pointed toward the ceiling. Inhale deeply.

2. On the exhale, begin to lower your head toward the ground, one vertebra at a time. Try to touch your hands to the floor.

3. Let your buttocks down toward the ground and, as you inhale, slowly allow your body to assume a squatting poition.

4. Hold this squat for as long as you can.

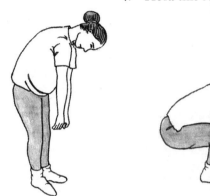 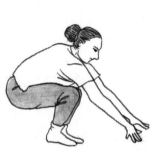 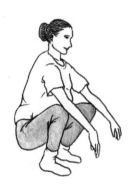

Cat Stretch

1. Start in a hands-and-knees position with your back parallel to the floor.

2. Exhale, drop your bely toward the floor.

3. Inhale, arching your back like a cat.

4. Repeat this sequence up to 20 times, following a gentle breathing rhythm.

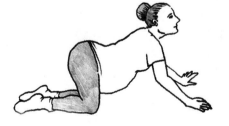 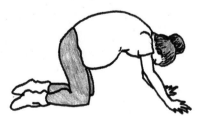

Forward Bend

1. Sitting upright on the floor, extend your legs to the sides, keeping them straight. Inhale deeply.

2. Exhaling, slowly lean forward, bringing your belly and chest as close to the floor in front of you as possible.

3. Inhale, sitting up straight, maintaining the leg position.

4. Repeat up to 10 times, getting closer to the floor the more you practice, and holding the forward bend longer.

5. Try alternating bending forward over each individual leg.

Butterfly Pose

1. Sit upright on the floor, flat on your buttocks.

2. With your legs bent at the knees and open to the sides, bring the soles of your feet together.

3. Holding on to your feet with your hands, draw your heels as close to your crotch as possible.

4. Gently 'flutter' your knees up and down, gradually bringing your knees closer to the floor.

5. Accompany this exercise with gentle inhalations and exhalations.

6. Maintain this pose for a little longer each session. Draw your feet in further and bring your knees closer to the ground for increasing difficulty.

7. Optional: You can try to touch your head to your feet for an added stretch to your inner thighs. Do not try to flutter your legs while doing this.

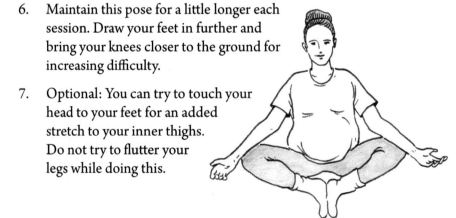

The Side-to-Side Stretch

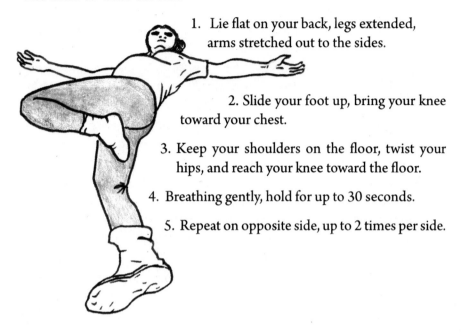

1. Lie flat on your back, legs extended, arms stretched out to the sides.

2. Slide your foot up, bring your knee toward your chest.

3. Keep your shoulders on the floor, twist your hips, and reach your knee toward the floor.

4. Breathing gently, hold for up to 30 seconds.

5. Repeat on opposite side, up to 2 times per side.

Leg Extensions

1. In a hands-and-knees position, gently lift your leg backward and upward, reaching toward the ceiling.

2. Return your knee to the floor.

3. Repeat up to 20 times, then repeat with the opposite leg.

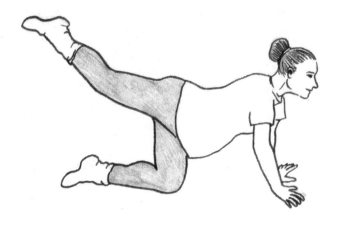

Birth Story: Ibu (Mother) Lina....

Was expecting her second baby. Her first pregnancy and birth were totally normal. This time, when she was seven weeks pregnant she reported to the midwife that there was bright red spotting. Her midwife took her to see Dr. Gabriel. Together Lina, her husband, and her midwife could see that the placenta was previa. This means the placenta is low-lying in the uterus, in this case it was so low that it was covering the cervix, which was causing the bleeding.

This was not good news, as if the placenta is covering the cervical opening at the time of birth a cesarean is necessary, because the placenta must never be born before the baby.

Lina's midwife had done a lot of reading about the miraculous placenta. "I have an idea," she said. "Let's talk to the placenta: Involve your entire family, and all the midwives in our practice. Together we can ask this placenta to migrate up north, out of the way of the cervix." This is an example of what can be called, "The biology of belief."

"Ok." said Dr. Gabriel, "We will try this intention and prayer experiment together." They agreed that Lina must take full bed rest and abstain from sexual relations for three weeks, or more, until all signs of bleeding have stopped. After that she may resume gentle activities, but no lifting. If everything went well, Lina could simply continue her regular prenatal check-ups with her midwife. They would meet again, with Dr. Gabriel, when Lina reached eight and a half months of pregnancy aka 38 weeks, to determine by ultra sound scan where the placenta was lying.

Well, the rest of Lina's pregnancy went well. There were no more incidents of bleeding. At eight and a half months Lina, her husband and her midwife went to see Dr. Gabriel. He looked worried, he did not want to give them bad news, but he had never seen a full placenta previa end in normal birth.

When they all looked inside of Lina's uterus, to find the position of the placenta, using the ultrasound machine, they were surprised. Dr. Gabriel shouted for joy and jumped up, for he could not believe his own eyes. He checked again and said. "It's a miracle! This placenta has moved all the way up and is clearly not in the way. You may have a normal natural birth Mother Lina.

"I wish to have a waterbirth this time," she said.

"I think that's a wonderful idea!" laughed her doctor. Two weeks later with the help of that same midwife at the birth center, in a pool of flowers and warm water, Lina birthed her son, Edi.

Ultrasound Issues

Some doctors, who specialized in obstetrics and gynecology, depend upon doing an ultrasound scan with every prenatal visit. There is research that says this is not necessary and not particularly healthy for the baby. Some mothers report that during ultrasound the baby inside was responding in a way that indicated she or he did not like the scan. You may decide not to have scans, if you feel uncomfortable with many unnecessary ultrasound examinations (also called sonogram). When you see a midwife for your regular prenatal pregnancy check ups, she will check you gently, without using an ultrasound machine. If she senses or finds a potential problem, she will recommend that you see a specialist Obgyn doctor, or Ultrasound technician, to get a scan. Your midwife will want to come along, or, look at the notes from the doctor, or speak with him or her, after your scan. In this way she can see what the results are and help you make wise decisions about your pregnancy and birth plans.

Sometimes women become afraid after ultrasound scans, for example, at less than 30 weeks of gestation your doctor may say, "Your baby is breech." Do not be alarmed, before 30 weeks breech presentation or position of baby is normal. Don't panic if your doctor tells you the baby is breech that early, in most cases the baby will naturally turn head down by 30 to 32 weeks. There are gentle exercises you can do to encourage the baby to move into a head down position. Sholat sujud position (praying Muslim style, hands-and-knees with your head lower than your behind) is one way to help the baby find a normal position. Hands and knees lifting and rounding your back, while tucking your buttocks pose, also known as "Cat~Cow" can help encourage the breech baby to go head down. Cleaning the floor on hands and knees, or laying on your back with your butt elevated on pillows, all help the baby find his or her way to a good birth position. Talk to baby, ask him or her to: move head down, tuck her chin and face your spine. Simply say, "Head down little one, tuck your chin, look at my back and put your hands on your heart." Your baby is listening!

If during an ultrasound scan your doctor makes the comment, "Your baby's umbilical cord is around her neck", please don't worry.

During your labor, the midwife will listen to baby's heartbeat regularly, to watch for signs of distress. Cord around the neck does not necessarily mean you must have a cesarean birth. About 20% of baby's born naturally, vaginally, have cord around the neck, and are just fine. The trick is to grow a long strong umbilical cord. You can do this, by following these simple tips.

Tips to grow a long umbilical cord with your baby...

Know that umbilical cords can gain much length, even in the last trimester of pregnancy. Eating lots of fruits and vegetables is standard advice for mothers who fear the baby will have a too short umbilical cord. Another common fear is that the cord is too tight around baby's neck. Again, the solution is feeding your body, the kinds of foods that will inspire the growth of a healthy long strong umbilical cord. I advise mothers to eat oranges and tangerines, selecting to eat the strings that lie along the inside of the citrus sections. Also, turn the peel inside out and eat the white part of the inside of the peel.

Talk to your baby's placenta, just as you speak to the baby. A low-lying placenta can be urged to migrate north, to the upper part of the uterus. Cords can get healthier and longer via good diet and prayerful intention. Remember, in Balinese culture the Placenta is the physical body of Baby's Guardian Angel, a protective soul. The placenta and the umbilical cord exist to help baby safely through gestation and birth.

Another ultra sound issue comes up when the doctor or Ultrasound Technician says: "You don't have enough amniotic fluid." In some countries, this leads to an automatic cesarean birth, for fear of undue strain on the baby and umbilical cord compression. Please don't be afraid. The first thing I suggest is: DRINK A LOT OF WATER! You can't get water into the amniotic sac with the baby, unless you take it into your body. The amniotic fluid does cushion the baby and support her during labor. Yes, it is important. If drinking a lot of water and/or young coconut water, does not increase your amniotic fluid try acupuncture and or homeopathy. I have seen both kinds of complimentary therapies really increase amniotic fluid, supporting normal vaginal gentle delivery.

If you are told you placenta is low lying in early pregnancy, please don't worry, as the uterus grows, placentas migrate up to the Northern regions of your uterus. Also, talk to your baby's placenta, he or she (genetically identical to baby) is an Angel whose soul purpose is to help Baby and Mother. Ask Placenta Angel to guard and protect Baby's health, and move to the best position for a gentle birth.

Ultrasound - How necessary? When? How often? These are questions that you may feel comfortable asking your midwife. She probably has a good relationship with a good back-up Obgyn doctor, who she will recommend, one who believes in the natural birth process, and will not try to find a reason for you to be afraid and have a cesarean birth unless you really need one.

Remember, you wish for Prenatal Care NOT Prenatal Scare!

*"I believe every woman has the right to
any birth experience she wants, wherever she chooses
and with whatever care provider she's comfortable.
It's about doing your own due diligence
and finding the best option for you."*

~ Ricki Lake

Prenatal Testing

First, if you are not sure your have conceived, you will have a pregnancy test, to detect the presence of hCG (Human Chorionic Gonadotrophin, which is a hormone released by a fertilized ovum). Congratulations if you are positive!

In most countries the expectant mother is offered, or told she must have many kinds of prenatal tests. Some of them make sense, and all mothers really should have some basic routine tests as a part of prenatal care. These include the routine checking/monitoring of:

- **Blood pressure,** to rule out pregnancy induced hypertension and preeclampsia. If it is high-ish in early pregnancy, you can immediately make better food and exercise choices, to normalize your blood pressure.

- **Weight ~ gain or loss.** Your midwife will want to know the baby is growing and your weight is increasing normally to account for increased blood volume, placenta and amniotic fluid, which all weigh something. You should gain weight, chronic loss of weight can signal that there are issues that need to looked at.

- **Measurement of Fundal Height,** also to determine if baby is growing.

- **Urine analysis** to test for a panel of things, ie blood or sugar or protein in urine, etc.

Non Routine Tests ~ Usually done... Recommended:

- **Complete Blood Count (CBC),** usually done once and sometimes twice in pregnancy, unless needed more often. Requires the drawing of a few CCs of mother's blood.

- **Tests for sexually transmitted infections,** usually done once, unless high risk behavior is reported by you, then the tests should be repeated. This is a good idea, because it is best for your baby if sexually transmitted infections are detected and cured, as early as possible. Usually this is done simultaneously with the Complete Blood Count.

- **Blood type, needed only once.** Done simultaneously with the CBC.

- **If your blood type is Rh-** and your baby's father is Rh+, you will wish to check your coombs, to know if you have been isoimmunized (sensitized against Rh+ blood. if this is the case your midwife and or doctor can advise you.

- **Check titers for rubella,** done once, usually this is done simultaneously with the Complete Blood Count.

- **Glucose tests to see if you have elevated blood sugar** should be done, if you have risks, ie family history, excessive weight gain, swelling, elevated blood pressure, slow healing of cuts.

- **GBS Group B Streptococcus tests** for GBS bacteria. GBS can cause serious infections leading to premature labor, infections of the placenta tissue, and postpartum infection. Risks for newborn include pneumonia and meningitis. Therefore it is recommended that pregnant mothers have a vaginal and rectal screening for GBS between 35 and 37 weeks gestation.

- **Ultrasound scan/screen** (also optional, especially if all is well with your pregnancy, I personally never had even one ultrasound when I was pregnant with my 5 babies.) Ultrasound is done to help determine baby's position (though in later pregnancy a good midwife or Obgyn can palpate your belly to determine baby's position). Ultrasound can determine if you are carry twins or triplets! A skilled Ultrasound technician (maybe a doctor or midwife too) will determine where your baby's placenta is, if baby's heart has four chambers, will look at baby's kidneys, and measure baby's head circumference, belly circumference, and femur length, to give a close approximation of gestational age. This can help determine your estimated date of delivery, even if you have forgotten your last monthly moon (period).

Tests Offered, but Not Necessary:

(meaning goblins will not take your baby away if you don't do these)~ You may ask yourself: "What will I do with the information, if I am told my baby may have special challenges?" If your answer is… you would do nothing, but allow your pregnancy to take it's course, then perhaps it's nice to not have these tests.

What Is A Screening Test?

Screening tests estimate what a person's chances are of having a special needs or unwell baby. Screening tests DO NOT diagnose a problem; they only signal if further testing will be recommended.

A diagnostic Test – Determines for sure, absolutely, that there is a genetic or health related irregularity. These things will be considered when prenatal screening and diagnostic tests are being offered:

- Age
- Ethnicity
- Results from earlier blood tests
- Family history of genetic irregularities

Nuchal transluncency (NT) Scan, Nuchal translucency is a collection of fluid under the skin at the back of your baby's neck, the scan to measure this fluid is done between 11 to 13 weeks after is meant to determine if the baby is alive and growing. Also, this scan is used to screen for possibility of Downs syndrome. This test is done by abdominal ultra sound, but sometimes to get accurate results a vaginal ultrasound scan is done. This means, if you agree or want this test, an ultrasound transducer will be put inside of your vagina. The ultrasound technician or doctor will measure the length from the crown of baby's head to the rump (butt), this is called the CRL. CRL is recognized as the most accurate way determine the baby's gestational age, and determine probable date of the birth. This test is most accurate if done before week 13 gestation.

At the same time the baby's Nuchal Translucency is checked to rule out the risk of Downs Syndrome.

1st Trimester biochemistry blood test is offered at the same time as NT Scan. A small sample of your blood is collected in order to do two biochemical tests on hormones being produced by the placenta. If these hormones are favorable, it indicates a reduced risk for your baby having Downs Syndrome.

The Triple Screening:
Pros

- The triple screen test is not invasive - blood is drawn from the mother.
- There are no known risks or side effects for baby, associated with the triple screen test.
- The results usually take a few days to receive.

Cons

- The triple screen test is known to have a high percentage of false positive results.

When Is The Triple Screen Test Done? 16th -18th week is the most accurate. It is recommended for women who:

- Have a family history of babies with special challenges ie genetic irregularities.
- If you are 35 years or older (never allow your doctor to scare you by calling your pregnancy a "Geriatric Pregnancy"!)
- If you used possible harmful medications or drugs during pregnancy
- If you have diabetes and use insulin
- If you had a viral infection during pregnancy
- If you have been exposed to high levels of radiation

What Does The Triple Screen Test Look For?
The triple screen is measuring high and low levels of AFP and abnormal levels of hCG and estriol.

High levels of AFP may suggest the developing baby has a neural tube defect such as spina bifida or anencephaly. However, the most common reason for elevated AFP levels is inaccurate dating of the pregnancy.

Low levels of AFP and abnormal levels of hCG and estriol may indicate that the developing baby has Trisomy 21 (Down Syndrome), Trisomy 18 (Edwards Syndrome) or another type of chromosome abnormality.

Although the primary reason for conducting the test is to screen for genetic disorders, the results of the triple screen can also be used to identify:

- A multiples pregnancy (twins or triplets)
- Pregnancies that are more or less advanced than you thought

What Do The Triple Test Results Mean?

This test only notes that a mother is at a possible risk of carrying a baby with a genetic disorder. Once you have abnormal test results then additional testing is recommended to make a diagnosis, such as:

- A second triple screen followed by a high definition ultrasound.
- If the testing still maintains abnormal results, a more invasive procedure like amniocentesis may be recommended. Invasive testing procedures should be discussed thoroughly with your healthcare provider and between you and your partner.
- Additional counseling and discussions with a counselor, social worker or a religious counselor, or minister may prove helpful.

What Are The Reasons For Further Testing?

Performing further testing allows you to confirm a diagnosis and then provides you with certain opportunities:

- To pursue potential interventions that may exist (i.e. fetal surgery for spina bifida)
- Begin planning for a child with special needs
- Start addressing anticipated lifestyle changes
- Identify support groups and resources
- Make a decision about carrying the child to term, or not
- Some individuals or couples may elect not to pursue testing or additional testing for various reasons:
- They are comfortable with the results no matter what the outcome is
- Because of personal, moral, or religious reasons, making a decision about carrying the child to term is not an option
- Some parents choose not to allow any testing that poses any risk of harming the developing baby

CVS Chorionic Villus Sampling is a diagnostic test of the baby's Chorionic sac. Baby placenta and amniotic fluid is double bagged in 2 sacs, the amnion, nearest to the baby, and the Chorion, the outer sac. It is a diagnostic test for identifying chromosome abnormalities and other inherited disorders like cystic fibrosis. CVS is an alternative to amniocentesis. It is very invasive as it requires removing a small amount of tissue called the chorionic villi, from outside the fetal gestational sac. (ouch) This is used for diagnostically for chromosome analysis but it cannot determine if the baby has neural tube defects. There are two ways samples are collected:

- **Transcervical:** An ultrasound guides a thin catheter through the cervix to your placenta. The chorionic villi cells are gently suctioned into the catheter. This is the most common method.

- **Transabdominal:** An ultrasound guides a long thin needle through the abdomen to your placenta. The needle draws a sample of tissue and then is removed. This procedure is similar to that of amniocentesis.

CVS is usually done between 10 and 13 weeks from your last moon, or menstrual period. CVS may be chosen over amniocentesis because it may be performed earlier in the pregnancy.

CVS Risks ~ Although CVS is considered by many doctors to be a safe procedure, it is recognized as an invasive diagnostic test that does pose potential risks. Miscarriage is the primary risk of CVS occurring 1 out of every 100 procedures.

CVS is not recommended for women who:
- Have an active infection (i.e. STI)
- Are carrying twins
- If you have had vaginal bleeding during this pregnancy

Transcervical CVS is not recommended for women who:
- Have a tilted uterus which could stop the catheter from easily entering your uterus
- Have uterine fibroids

Following the procedure, the mother may experience one or more of the following side effects. Contact your healthcare provider if you experience these symptoms.:

- Infection
- Spotting
- Cramping and pain at puncture point

You should also contact your healthcare provider if you experience:

- Fever
- Intense Nausea
- Chills
- Leaking of amniotic fluid

According to the Mayo Clinic, there is a 1% chance of getting false positive results. A false positive occurs when the test indicates that the fetus has an abnormality, but it actually does not.

Amniocentesis is a diagnostic test in which a thin needle is guided through your abdomen into the baby's amniotic sac, in order to obtain a sample of baby's amniotic fluid. Fetal cells gathered are used for chromosome tests and specific genetic testing, to determine if your baby is at risk for Down syndrome and other chromosome or gestational irregularities. It is very invasive. It will be recommended if the results of earlier test, like the Triple Screen are deeded unfavorable. It is usually done between 14 and 20 weeks gestation. Amniocentesis is occasionally used late in pregnancy to assess whether the baby's lungs are mature enough for the baby to breathe on his own, only if the doctors are considering early delivery of the baby. Your doctor may recommend the procedure if your membranes have ruptured prematurely, in order to assess for uterine infections. Amniocentesis may also help determine the severity of fetal anemia in babies with Rh disease (sensitized Rh- mom and Rh+ baby), and assist your physician determine whether the fetus requires blood transfusions.

Amniocentesis detects:

- Chromosome abnormalities - Down's syndrome
- Neural tube defects – spina bifida
- Genetic disorders – cystic fibrosis
- Paternity testing – The results are 99% accurate

What Are The Risks?

Miscarriage is the primary risk related to amniocentesis. And occurs 1 in 400 to 1 in 200 depending of the skills of the person doing it. Miscarriages can occur because of:

- Infection in the uterus
- Water breaking
- Labor being induced prematurely

Anatomy Ultrasound or Level II testing is offered at 18 to 20 weeks to survey the baby's anatomy, to check for irregularities and to see if baby is growing correctly. If you do not wish to know the sex of your baby, make it clear before this ultrasound scan begins, or the technician and/or doctor may just tell you, like it our not!

When deciding weather to have or not to have certain prenatal tests, ask yourself; "What will I do with this information? If my baby was found to have some congenital irregularities, would I terminate this pregnancy? Would having these tests lower or heighten my stress level?" Some parents wish to know if a Baby has challenges, even if they do not wish to terminate. This can help them plan for the Baby's special needs, before his or her arrival.

These are hard questions. The answers must be found by you and your partner, if you have one, delving deep into your own inner knowing. Every MotherBabyFamily is different, some wish to know all they can, others wish to keep the mystery of the miracle of sexual reproduction. No one must judge.

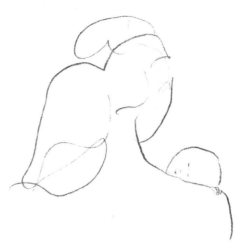

"My second daughter was born with Down Syndrome. Though I had all the tests, and none of them showed risks for trisomy 21 or other congenital issues. Because all of the early tests were clear, my husband and I decided not to have amniocentesis. We are so happy we did not do this more conclusive test. We feel our child, with all her challenges is perfect, just the way she is. We do not regret having her. We don't wish she were different. She is our daughter, and we feel blessed."

~ *Katelynn, mother of two*

"Since I was 37 years old, my doctor convinced me to have amniocentesis, though I don't think I would have aborted my baby, if the tests showed risks. It took my husband and I eight years of trying to finally achieve pregnancy, we were so happy. The amniocentesis proved my baby was forming perfectly and had no chromosome damage, or congenital abnormalities. Tragically, an infection began, as a side effect of the invasion of the amniocentesis needle into our baby's amniotic sac. This infection caused a miscarriage, and we lost our tiny son.

I was blessed to become pregnant again, less than a year later, though I was still grieving. My husband and I refused all tests, and we have a beautiful healthy daughter."

~ *Mia, finally a mother*

Pregnancy over 35

Author's note: I have had mothers come to me, crying because a doctor told them they were carrying a "Geriatric Pregnancy" because they were 35 years or older. This is just mean! Some mothers who are more mature physically, may wish to get all the prenatal screening and testing, others may opt for some screening, and others none at all. Most Obgyns and some midwives recommend prenatal screening especially for mothers who are over 35 years of age. Remember, you have a right to kind, RESPECTFUL prenatal care (not prenatal scare). This is your body, your baby. You have a right to information that can help you make the wisest decisions for your baby and for you.

Remember, many observations and assumptions about the risks of pregnancy over the age of 35 years, were made decades ago, when women had less information on how to stay healthy. Many women well over the age of 40 enjoy perfect health and fertility. Being mature does not mean you will have a baby with problems. Worrying and being afraid is not good for you or your baby.

My own mother was a 9th child, born when my Filipino Lola was forty-four years old. Two years later, at the age of forty-six, my Lola had her last baby, my Auntie Isabel. These perfectly healthy women now in their mid-eighties, were born naturally, gently, into the hands of traditional midwives, at home, in the 1930s.

Affirmations...

"I have ample courage to face these amazing changes in my life."

"Baby, thank you for kicking, rolling, dancing and playing soccer in there... letting me know just how ALIVE we are together."

"Baby... I trust that you are with me, designing a perfect birth plan for both of us."

What if my Baby is Breech?

Some mothers get afraid if, after an ultrasound, they are told their baby is breech in early pregnancy. It is quite normal for babies to still be head-up when you are 29 to 30 weeks pregnant and then to turn head-down around 32 to 34 weeks gestation. Some doctors may be concerned if, at 36 weeks along, your baby is still head-up. Most midwives will not worry, but will give you the kind of guidelines that I am going to share now, to help your baby choose the head-down position.

My second baby, Noel, who is now 36 years old and a wonderful dad, was in the breech position until just two days before he was born, at 39 weeks gestation. Looking back, my midwives may have been concerned, but they did not let on. Mary and Debbie calmly instructed me in the breech tilt position. It worked.

Breech Tilt:

Comfortably lay on the floor with one or two pillows under your butt. Make sure your bladder is empty. Put your hands and attention on the baby, talk to her or him... "Baby, I need you to turn your head down, so our birth will be easier. Tuck your chin, baby... put our hands on your heart, let your head move down into my pelvis and look at my spine." Do this 3 times per day for about 4 to 5 minutes. You would be surprised at how often this alone works wonderfully.

Knee to Chest ~ or Sholat Prayer Position:

Also very effective, alternate with the Breech Tilt position.

When the baby moves head-down, it can feel like a small earthquake inside. This is what I felt when my breech baby finally put his head down. I called my midwives and they invited me over, so that they could confirm what I felt. Yes... Baby was vertex! Two days later, he was born after a 2 ½ hour labor!

Note: You may wish to consult a Homeopathic physician, sometimes taking homeopathic Pulsatilla 30c, before doing the Breech Tilt, can make it more effective.

One of the most effective ways to turn a breech baby is via acupuncture. Doctors of Traditional Chinese Medicine are learned in how to naturally coax babies into optimal position for birth. It normally takes two to three visits to the doctor of TCM, before the baby is convinced to turn. Even if baby does not turn head-down, the acupuncture prepares mOms for birth, postpartum and breastfeeding.

My grandmother, Vicenta Munar Lim, was skilled at gentle massage to turn breech babies, like many traditional Hilots in the Philippines and Dukun Bayi in Indonesia once were. I have some skill, in doing the external breech version. When I lay my hands upon the belly of a mother carrying a breech baby, I say a silent prayer to Divine Mother and to the Baby, asking permission to go ahead, mostly I get a strong feeling of "YES." If I do not, I won't attempt to turn that baby with my hands.

Once Baby has moved into head-down position, I like to wrap the mother's belly, and help her to walk up and down stairs, so the baby engages vertex, and is ready for birth.

The Question of Due Dates

Some women have long menstrual cycles others have short cycles, this will also determine your due date, not just the calendar. Do not jump to the conclusion your baby is late, especially if your menstrual cycles are long, for example over 31 days. (Count the days of your cycle from first day of moon or bleeding to last day before onset of next menstruation.) Mothers with short cycles, under 27 days, may have their babies sooner than mothers with more average length cycles of 28 to 31 days.

Many times I have answered the phone in the night to find a mother weeping on the line. Why? Because she is not due for several more days, and her contractions have begun, or her waters have released. When I explain that this must be the Baby's birthday, and it's perfectly ok for birth to happen when Baby is ready, not when the calendar prescribes, these mothers sigh with relief.

Dating by ultrasound aka sonogram, is it correct? Ultrasound due date determination done in the early weeks of pregnancy is often quite accurate. However, late in pregnancy ultrasound due date determination can be close but not perfectly accurate. If your ultra sound practitioner is very skilled and experienced, then the estimated date of delivery will be more accurate. Stress, worry, pressure, can all speed up or more likely delay the onset of true labor.

Babies generally come when they are ready, just as the ripe fruit falls easily from the tree. Being one week "late" is not a problem, worrying is a sure way to make your baby come even later. If you are one week or even two or more weeks past your calendar due date and your doctor says you need a cesarean, get another opinion to determine if there are true risk factors indicating the need for surgical birth. (Remember what we said about choosing a doctor who has a very low rate of cesareans.) Generally midwives are not worried unless the baby is more than 2 to 3 weeks later than the calendar due date, for a woman with short or average cycles. In this case she may ask you to have an ultrasound scan with a good doctor, who believes in natural childbirth. The doctor will look at the amount of amniotic fluid, position of baby and evaluate your heath, to help you make wise decisions. It is important that you are drinking plenty of pure water, so that you will have plenty of amniotic fluid to cushion the baby's way. The doctor will also observe with ultrasound the position and condition of the placenta. The baby's movements will also be observed. If all is well, and the doctor is fair, you will be advised to wait for your labor to begin naturally.

Women with long cycles, for example 35 days or more, your baby may well stay inside past the due date you were given, please do not worry. If you must worry, give yourself a 5 to 15 minute "worry spell." Then offer it up to the Baby's Angels, and go about your day.

Does making love get labor going?

Sometimes gentle loving sex can inspire labor to begin. This is only advised if you are not leaking amniotic fluid. You and your husband should be free of sexually transmutable diseases. The two of you can find a comfortable, side-lying position to gently make love. The prostaglandin hormones in your husband's semen helps to soften the cervix and get you ready for labor. The pleasure you feel will stimulate the uterine contractions you need to begin labor naturally. The love hormone, oxytocin will make it unfold as nature intended it.

I believe the Baby actually gives the green light for the onset of labor. When his or her parents are joined in gentle lovemaking, the baby just may feel it's safe to come out join our world.

It is quite normal to be afraid of labor beginning. When making love you may find it a good time to talk about this fear with your husband, even have a good cry. All of this helps soften your spirit and your body into naturally and gently going into labor. Before each of my labors began, I had a good cry.

A Nice "Due Date" affirmation:

Mother Nature and Father Time, working for the Divine Creator, are resonating with my Baby's soul. Together they will know when my Baby is ready to be born not when doctors, midwives or anyone else decides. My baby will be born healthy, at the perfect time.

Story of ADE...

Ade and Wayan's first baby was a 4 kilogram boy. He was born naturally after about 18 hours of labor, at Bumi Sehat, in the care of midwives.

When Ade was expecting her second baby, two and a half years later, she felt good. She went regularly to the midwives at the Bumi Sehat Bali Birth Center for check ups, she ate well, drank plenty of pure water and enjoyed fresh orange juice often. She also took her prenatal vitamins.

As it sometimes happens, Ade's baby did not come on her calendar due date. This did not surprise her, as her first son was born nine days "late". Because Ade's menstrual cycles were not regular and were often long, the midwives had assured her that her baby was not really "late".

Ade's husband's boss became concerned because Ade was six days past her "due date." She meant well, but she pressured Ade and Wayan into seeing her doctor in the city for an ultrasound scan. Ade had been seeing the same Obgyn doctor she and her midwife trusted, but was too shy to refuse her husband's bosses' attempt to be helpful.

The new doctor really tried to frighten Ade and Wayan and their friend. He said, "The amniotic fluid is nearly non-existent. The baby is so late that he has shrunken in the womb. The placenta is calcified and small, no longer supporting the baby's life. The cord is wrapped dangerously around the baby's neck two times. The baby's heartbeat is dangerously slow. You must immediately have a cesarean, or your baby will die!"

These words frightened everyone. However, Ade tuned into her own mothering instincts. She bravely told the doctor, "If my baby was in so much danger, why don't I FEEL it?" She refused the cesarean, and went that same evening, with her midwife, and her now terrified husband to see her original trusted Obgyn doctor. He said, "Your baby is very big and fat, like your first one! There is plenty of amniotic fluid. Your baby's heartbeat is perfect, as is the placenta. I find no cord around the neck. Yes, you are about one week late by your calendar dates, but that feels normal for you, Ade. My advice to you is to go home, eat a nice dinner together, rest, and make juicy love. I just bet you will go into labor by morning." He turned to the midwife, "Call me when the baby is safely born. I think it will be just fine. Of course, if there are complications, you can call me for help, anytime, that's what I'm here for."

Ade and Wayan went home, they followed the Doctor's wise instructions. In the morning Ade woke up in good strong labor. They rushed over to Bumi Sehat Birth Center, where the Midwives had the waterbirth tub filled and waiting. Ade had a lovely natural waterbirth, no complications. The doctor was so happy to hear the news. They never saw the other doctor again, but they wondered why he lied to them.

Ade was laughing when her baby was born, a healthy 5 kilo girl!

The story of Ade is a perfect example why it is important to choose a midwife, or a group of midwives who work together, who care about you and who have a personal touch when it comes to your prenatal care. Your Midwives should also have a good relationship with one or more skilled doctors, who believe in gentle childbirth, and who believe in women's ability to birth naturally. Ade would have succumbed to an unnecessary cesarean birth, had she not believed in and listened to her own inner knowing. Well done Ibu Ade!

Taking Castor Oil to Induce Labor...

Note: Only do this supervised by your midwife and/or doctor.

Sometimes castor oil induction is used to inspire labor if you have gone more than 2 weeks beyond your estimated due date. Remember due dates are estimates, IF the baby is not ready and you do castor oil, you will have wicked diarrhea and even intense cramping, but not true labor. No cervical dilation will occur.

If you have premature rupture of the amniotic/chorionic membranes PROM, and your baby's amniotic fluid has released, labor will usually begin on it's own, within a few hours. Care should be taken to prevent the invasion of bacteria into your womb, as Baby is no longer sealed in an impenetrable double walled sac. NO tub baths, NO love making, penetration of your vagina with anything is to be absolutely avoided, to thwart infection. Midwives often avoid even doing a vaginal exam to determine if some dilation has occurred. If she does a vaginal exam it will be done in a strictly sterile procedure. Mothers with PROM should be careful on the toilet to only wipe from front to back. Strict hygiene must be kept once PROM has occurred.

If labor does not begin on it's own after PROM, then a natural induction with castor oil may be done by your midwife or doctor.

The mother should only be advised to have castor oil, under the supervision of a skilled birth attendant (midwife). Mother should be well rested, castor oil induction is best begun in the early morning after a good night's sleep. The cervix must be ripe. Prior to drinking castor oil the MotherBaby should be checked to see that the baby's heartbeat is normal. The midwife will palpate to check for the baby's position. Mother's blood pressure and physical/mental/emotional bodies will be evaluated. Each midwife has her preferred recipe for effective use of castor oil to stimulate labor. Please, don't just decide you are finished with this pregnancy, and want to get the labor going. Some mothers just go on the internet and find a recipe for castor oil induction, that is not a safe way to do it. Talk to your midwife, please.

Some other suggested methods of natural labor stimulation are: nipple stimulation, a good foot and body massage, eating spicy/oily foods, ie add a lot of spicy peanut sauce to your favorite dish! Sometimes a good cry, a long wonderful walk in nature... can stimulate labor to begin. Making love can really begin labor, if mother and baby are both ready. Again remember, any penetration, genital to genital or hand genital contact must be strictly avoided after the amniotic fluid has leaked or gushed out.

Twins in Bali ~ Awakening Birth, Spiced with Global Drama

...or, the reluctant miracle

By Robin Lim & Deborah Flowers

A decision to support a mother who presents late in an atypical pregnancy is never something we do lightly at Bumi Sehat. BirthKeepers may find themselves walking a delicate line, between advocating for human rights in childbirth, and taking risks. While processing these kinds of decisions, both during and afterwards, it is good to stand firmly upon three feet: good skills/science, respect for nature, and "adat" which means spirit/faith/intuition. Also, it feels best to share responsibility with sister midwives, who resonate in practice and enhance one another's skills. Here Deborah Flowers, one of the Tennessee Farm Midwives, and I, endeavor to share a difficult decision, a good outcome, with some bumps along the way.

Olga a forty-four year old multi gravida, fled Russia, where she faced certain cesarean birth. Russian childbirth stories speak of cruelty in the delivery rooms and include a common practice in Moscow hospitals; keeping the babies isolated from family for the first 3 to 5 days of life. During this time, the parents cannot see the baby, nor can the mother breastfeed her baby. This, according to concerned Russian parents, is done to make sure the next generation of Russians cannot make deep human connections, by shattering each newborn baby's capacity to love and trust. In this way the prevailing government in power may prevent a future revolution. Clearly denying Babies and Mother their Sacred First Embrace has a profound negative effect on all society, all of our Earth.

Olga arrived at Bumi Sehat Bali 34 weeks pregnant, wearing dark circles under her tired eyes.

Her first visit was hugs and tears. Olga looked into the eyes of the Bumi Sehat *bidan-bidan* (midwives), and begged us, "Please cesarean, no."

Olga was accompanied to Bali by a Russian interpreter, Ilena, a blessing as Olga's English was minimal and she spoke no Bahasa Indonesia. Ilena was curious about all things concerning childbirth, as she had no experience with pregnancy and birth, at all.

Our Balinese midwives were astonished at the size if Olga's belly. We learned from Olga and Ilena that she was carrying twins. These babies would be Olga's forth and fifth children. Olga's husband, a truck driver, had saved diligently to send his wife to Bumi Sehat Bali, in desperation, to prevent more of the trauma his family had suffered when the first three children were born. He was home in Moscow, working, his parents looking after the 3 children who stayed behind.

When mothers-to-be from foreign lands, who live in Indonesia, seek care with us, we are happy to oblige. When foreign families write to us, wishing to come as tourists, to have their babies gently, we discourage them, because, should transport be necessary, the hospitals here are just not nice. The Neonatal intensive care units are always full and quite ineffective in saving newborns lives, when needed. I had a vague memory of Olga's husband writing to me, many weeks earlier. I advised them not to come to Bali, and did not hear from them again.

(The Bumi Sehat 2014/15 childbirth data shows a 2.4% transport for cesarean rate. Some of these cesarean births were not necessary, in our opinion, however if the laboring mother and her family request transport, we oblige and help them with free ambulance service and postpartum/breastfeeding support.)

At Bumi Sehat we do have ultrasound, however we do not use it routinely. Most of our mothers-to-be do not have ultrasound scans. In the case of Olga, she requested ultra sound to determine the positions of her twins, and we midwives agreed it was wise.

Olga's first coming twin was transverse, and through the amnions and chorions she (baby #1) was sucking on the knee of her breech brother! (Olga already knew the genders of her babies, otherwise we would have avoided noticing/revealing. I spoke with these babies, "Ok Twins… no more being naughty. Your mother wishes for you to have the most gentle birth, you need to tuck your little chins and turn head down." Olga laughed to hear this. What she did not know is that the Department of Health in Indonesia no longer allows midwives to handle twins, breech or VBAC births. At that moment I felt it was my duty to give Olga Prenatal CARE, not Prenatal SCARE. I really was not concerned that we would need to break regulations to do this birth, because at that moment, it seemed impossible, considering their positions. I underestimated this mother's clarity of intention and power to manifest her dream.

This gentle mother looked me in the eyes and expressed, with the help of her interpreter, "I want to have a gentle, homebirth (she was in a hotel), waterbirth (outlawed in Indonesia by "Pogi" the Obgyn association and DOH) and lotus birth (the doctors once willing to do cesarean lotus births stopped, as they faced loss of license!)."

I took a deep breath, hugged her and said, "Let's help your babies find their optimal birth position first. Ilena translating from English into Russian, I was translating from Russian into Indonesian, so all could be understood... all our BirthKeeper hearts were heavy, weighing the Mother's dream, with the reality of this twin pregnancy. Add to that the political climate surrounding birth in Indonesia.

At Bumi Sehat Bali we have acupuncture, homeopathy and holistic complimentary medicine, five mornings per week, for free. Olga attended acupuncture to turn her babies, plus got the Traditional Chinese Medicine treatments for "Happy Baby." (happy Baby treatments are meant to alleviate karma between mother and baby, babies in this case, to smooth the way for birth and beyond.) The holistic medicine team at Bumi Sehat made it their project to help Olga and the babies. We midwives taught her the breech tilt position and gave her homeopathic Pulsatilla 30c, to take before her routine of breech tilt two or three times per day, for a few minutes. Olga also joined our prenatal yoga class, three days per week, where she became friends with many Indonesian mothers-to-be. She wore a genuine smile, a mother on a mission.

Olga also wished to consult an obgyn, we recommended one who resonates with the Gentle Birth vision. He advised her to have a cesarean, unless both babies turn head down.

By the end of Olga's 36th week of pregnancy, baby #1 was head down. Baby #2 was transverse. More acupuncture, healthy eating, prenatal yoga, homeopathy and doing breech tilt....

Week 37, baby #1 head down, Baby #2 was breech, knees down. Olga continued to eat very well, went for walks in the Monkey Forest, and came for acupuncture, prenatal yoga and prenatal care, with the Bumi Sehat midwives. Masha, a Russian midwife and Bumi Sehat mother, formed a deep friendship with Olga.

On the day Olga became 38 weeks, she came early for her prenatal check-up, both her babies were head down! She danced around the Bumi Sehat clinic, with her midwives. We all cried tears of joy. We were now feeling that there was no reason for Olga to plan a cesarean. However, the obgyn felt concerned that there was just "Too much Baby in there... not safe."

Olga decided that she felt safe and bonded to Bumi Sehat and the team of midwives. She would have her baby at the birth center, with midwives she had grown to love and trust. I was relieved, as I did not feel comfortable doing a homebirth for this Mother/Babies. I felt I needed the resources of the entire Bumi Sehat midwifery team.

The Bumi Sehat midwives felt blessed, because Deborah Flowers, one of the Tennessee Farm Midwives, with 33 years of experience as a BirthKeeper, was visiting. She had handled breech and twin births for decades. Her experience combined with the other two senior midwives, on the birth team that night, added up to over 85 years! Masha, our Russian midwife, would join us for Olga's birth, bringing her skills as an interpreter, a doula and a midwife.

We advised Olga to balance rest with activity, eat well, and ignore the "Prenatal Scare" she was getting at the obgyn's office. She asked for a vaginal exam, to determine if her cervix was ripe and effaced. I found her cervix not ripe, perhaps 30% effaced, and quite long and closed. All of Olga's children arrived about one week after her due dates (determined by Ultrasound and calendar). Midwife Masha and I assured her that these babies would begin the labor on just the right day or night, already determined on the Divine Creator's calendar, but not known to us... yet.

2 nights later, Olga and her translator arrived at Bumi Sehat. She was having intense contractions, and pooing heaps of watery diarrhea. We advised her to drink but this was difficult, as she did not want to take anything by mouth. Still we pushed oral fluids, and Olga tried to do her best.

"Did you take castor oil?" I asked. Ilena, the interpreter looked sideways at Olga, and blurted out, "Yes, she took 120 ml four hours ago, that's how this labor began." I tried not to make a sound, just supportive back rubs were in order, but I was not happy. Outside Midwives, Wayan, Masha, Deborah and I, shook our heads, wishing that this labor had been allowed to begin without the castor oil push, and such a big dose of castor oil.

All of the Bumi Sehat midwives use castor oil quite conservatively. IF there is a real need, i.e., premature rupture of membranes and doctor threatening cesarean just 6 hours later, or going three weeks past due date, again, only because the mother is threatened with cesarean by the next day. Before using castor oil we feel the mother must have had a good night's sleep. We start castor oil inductions in the early morning, so everyone on the team is well rested. The cervix must be ripe and the baby's heart rate must be strong and perfect. Olga had asked me to induce her with castor oil a couple of days earlier, I felt is was a better idea to wait and allow the babies to initiate labor. I worried that the first coming baby may be ready, but the second coming, smaller baby, may just need some more days, even a couple of weeks to cook.

The castor oil made Olga's labor very uncomfortable. She was on the toilet so much. At Bumi Sehat the toilets are the typical Asian style squat toilets, which Olga found challenging while in labor. We were concerned about dehydration, and Olga said she was exhausted. This was not turning out to be the gentle birth she had wished for. The under-ripe cervix, was opening ever so stubbornly, it was many hours of work for Olga, with our continuous support and care.

Suddenly Olga was having a strong urge to push. She asked to be checked. She also told us her doctor in Russia said, "You cannot have your babies, unless we break the water bag." Midwife Wayan, Deborah, Masha, and I, all felt it would be unwise to rupture the amnion and chorion, to release the waters. With these twins, we felt Mother Nature and Father Time plus the Babies... would lead us along the safest road. We did check Olga, She was 7 to 8 cm, with the 1st coming baby very low in her pelvis, almost on-view, with bulging amniotic sac.

The next contraction, Olga rolled off of the low bed, into a squat, she was pushing. "Oh..." says Midwife Deborah, "We've got a head here." and she received that Baby.

What came next was unmitigated jubilation, which included Mother Olga jumping around quite rapidly, holding the Baby up-high, we were even worried that the umbilical cord would break! The interpreter was terrified by everything that she had seen, and was in the corner, unavailable to help us explain to Olga. We needed Olga to calm down and allow us to hold the 2nd coming baby, in his head-down position. We needed to listen to his heartbeat. We needed to see the first baby, in mother's arms, was safe and well, insuring her intact umbilical cord was not being pulled too taut. I could hear Midwife Masha speaking firmly in Russian.

We midwives put our arms around Olga and at the same time brought the baby closer. Midwife Wayan had the Doppler and as Masha coaxed Olga into a calmer state, I tired to hold her 2nd coming twin in a good position, it was like trying to hold a mother tiger still, add heaps of slippery amniotic fluid, impossible chaos! Deborah and Wayan tried to listen with the doppler. When they finally found the 2nd twin's heartbeat, it was abnormally slow, dropping to 80 beats per minute, and 40 beats per minute. Too slow, Baby was floundering.

Contrary to how we normally practice, we got Olga to lay down, so we could better evaluate and make fast decisions. Listening again, the 2nd twin's heart rate was still plummeting. He would die, if we did not help him.

All the bouncing around, the yet unborn twin's position had shifted, he was no longer head down, ready for birth, he was transverse.

The terrible sound of the doppler rang in my ears. Deborah, Masha, Wayan and I were in a state of pure communication, I can't remember our words. Deborah remembers saying, "You need to break the water and go in, find the feet and bring him out." In that moment I knew Deborah was right, I would need to bring this distressed baby out, immediately.

Olga could not seem to understand that there was another baby to come. I had to get my hand inside of her, to release the amniotic waters, and extract the baby, fast. Had this been birth at a hospital, the 2nd baby would be removed by emergency cesarean. There was no time for a transport. We needed to act, clearly and with skill.

Widiya, our apprentice midwife, let us know it was now 18 minutes since the birth of the first twin. I made the decision to clamp and cut the umbilical cord, so I could work, and so Olga would focus on the next baby, and allow me to do what had to be done. Olga said, "Please no." she did not want her baby girl's cord severed.

Olga wished for Lotus Births for these twins, I also wished...
but at the moment, I felt I could not get Olga to focus on the birth of
her second twin, and allow me to work efficiently to remove her baby,
unless we moved the first twin from her arms. Also, the cord was now
white and limp, so we knew the baby had her full blood supply and
stem cells.

This is the part of this birth that disturbs me, I made a decision
that mother was not happy with. I felt I was making the decision in
the best interest of the 2nd twin. Looking back... I wonder IF I could
have just done the job at hand, with the 1st twin intact?

There was a moment of surrender from Olga, Midwife Wayan
clamped and cut the cord, Widiya held the baby, Deborah and Masha
held the mother tight, and kept her eyes locked to their own. I went
inside the mother's sacred deepest place. I found the transverse baby
very high up, it was a shock, to need to go in so deep. I felt for the
amniotic sac, it was tough, and I had to struggle to rupture it. The
water came in a big gush. I found the baby's feet, and brought him,
as gently and swiftly as I could, into the footling breech position and
he was born to the waste. Quickly his torso and one arm were born. I
asked for help. Midwives Deborah and Wayan, swiveled Olga to the
edge of the bed, so gravity would help the baby come right down tenderly. There was no time to hesitate, the moment the nape of his neck
showed us hair, Deborah and Wayan lifted him up, so his face would
clear the perineum.

Deborah: One thing that I remember was with Radomir (2nd
coming baby), after you (Ibu Robin) had him out to his waist and
then you got one arm out, you asked me to help. I was thinking that
because he was so much smaller than his sister, that it would be easy
to deliver the second arm and head and that if I lifted his feet the second arm would probably just come and that the head would follow,
so I started to do that. At that point Ibu Robin said, "Let's bring Mom
to the edge of the bed." I thought, "That will work too." Also there was
not a lot of time for discussion, so we brought Mom to the edge of the
bed to let baby dangle to see the nape of the neck. I went in and swept
his arm down right before we moved Mom. He came easily.

This baby boy was much smaller than his sister and he needed
help getting started. While the labor was going on, Widiya, had set up

the full neonatal resuscitation kit. The delee was used, Radomir was given a long opening breath with the bag and mask, and then another. Deborah took the oxygen tube from the mother's nose (put there when baby #2 went into distress), and gave some blow-by O2 to baby, while we determined his heart beat was rising, and we continued to use the bag and mask to help him breathe. Heart rate was so slow, Deborah was performing full neonatal resuscitation, with breaths and chest compressions. This baby's APGAR was 2 at 1 minute, and quickly improved to 7 by 10 minutes. Olga was soon breastfeeding her daughter, Milanda, with Widiya's help. Deborah continued to stimulate and monitor Radomir's recovery from his not-so-gentle landing.

Olga had only a small tear and she did not hemorrhage. She was sad that we clamped and cut her baby girl's cord, after only 18 minutes. I am sad too. Soon both the placentas were born, the membranes woven together. We left the Baby boy intact with the placentas, so he had a full lotus birth, as was his mother's wish. I apologized for putting my hand inside of her. I had asked Olga's permission, at the time. To be honest, I cannot recall if Olga had agreed, there was a language barrier. I believe that what I did was necessary to preserve the 2nd twin's life, but NOT at all gentle.

The baby boy had trouble latching and breastfeeding, as we sometimes see when a baby requires some suctioning and resuscitation. By dawn it was getting better, and he could get on his mother's breast to feed. He did not have the vigor that his twin sister had.

Many hours after the Babies were born, Olga shared her secret with us… that her 3rd baby was born by cesarean, because that baby was over 5 kilograms and the doctor in Russia was afraid that was just too much baby to birth safely, considering Olga had a history of postpartum hemorrhage after her first two births.

This baby boy weighed 2.900 kg while the girl was 4,100 kg, that's 7 kilos of baby, or 15.432 lbs! I had not noticed Olga's cesarean scar during prenatal care, there were lots of stretch marks, and from Olga's stories, shared in translation, I assumed all three of her previous births had been vaginal.

I honestly don't think we would have attempted this birth-out-of-hospital, had we known that Olga was a VBAC, with a history of postpartum hemorrhage.

After about 24 hours the baby boy was quite lethargic and yellow. Olga did not want to draw his blood to test his bilirubin, so we simply used the Bili Blanket, to do blue light therapy. Olga stayed skin-to-skin with her weaker baby, Radomir, breastfeeding him as continuously as possible during his 12 hours of blue light therapy. There was the other twin, Milanda, to feed and care for, all the Bumi Sehat midwives helped the mother to cope. Olga already had heaps of milk, a blessing. Subsequently, the baby girl also developed jaundice, and we used the Bili Blanket to give her blue light therapy, during the next 12 hours.

Our postpartum visits with Olga have been wonderful and loving, full of laughter and admiration for everyone involved. This mother's determination and positive temperament prevailed to bring her twins Earth-side in the most natural viable way. Olga indicates that she feels she had the best, most positive, respectful possible birth, far more satisfying, loving and awakened than all her other childbirth experiences.

Twins in Bali Deborah Flower's version

Mama: 5th pregnancy, 1 miscarriage, 2 vaginal births in Russia, 1 cesarean birth, 3 living children, no preterm babies, 5 living children including these twins.

Twin A – girl Milanda 9 lbs 4.1 kg vertex

Twin B – boy Radomir 6 ½ lbs 2.95 kg breech

Born May 8th 5 am and 5:22 am

The Mom is from Russia and came to Bumi Sehat to avoid a cesarean. She was tired of being pregnant and took castor oil without asking us, and she took it at 8pm and went right into labor, so we were up all night. Probably not the right thing for her to have done. I think that both babies could have cooked a bit more. Her three other children were all very large at birth and by ultra sound the twins were both vertex and large enough to be born, but not as large as her other children.

The Mom said that baby A, the girl always moved a lot when I was around so we decided that I'd catch her and Robin would catch baby B. Baby A came one push after SROM while Mom was squatting.

We got Mom back up on the bed and found that baby B had changed from vertex to transverse and his heart rate was dropping 108, 80, 40, 25. So we decided the best thing to do was to break the water and go get him by the feet and bring him out. Robin found his feet, she turned him to back up and pulled him down. Robin got one arm, I got the other arm and we brought the mother to the edge of the bed and let baby dangle and I delivered his head, with Bumi Sehat Midwife Wayan. It was a little intense to say the least. We gave him a 2/7 Apgar. The girl had an Apgar of 8/9.

They were supposed to be 38 weeks and 3 days but they were covered in vernix and grunting and retracting quite a lot. I was glad that I brought my flow-inflating bag, for neonatal resuscitation, on this trip, so I did some CPAP on both of them. Using pulse oximetry we checked their oxygen saturation and the girl (baby #1) was saturating oxygen well so I didn't worry about her grunting and by 3 or 4 hours of age she stopped. The boy's O2 saturation would drop to the 60s on room air, but he did well with a little blow by. I put a nasal cannula on him and at 1 LPM his oxygen saturation was 93 – 94.

I showed the Balinese midwives at the clinic how to check his O2 saturation and how much oxygen to give him and to call if anything changed. The NICUs here at the hospitals are often full and the care is inconsistent. From past experience of 25 years of living in Bali and working in Maternal and Infant healthcare, Robin believed that this baby had a better chance of living if we took care of him ourselves, than if we transported him. Had there been a dependable NICU, we surely would have brought this baby in.

I went to the clinic to check on the twins every few hours to be sure they were both doing well and to be sure that baby B was doing ok on the nasal cannula. I almost got Baby B weaned off oxygen when he was 10 hours old, but had to put him back on 0.5 LPM, to keep his O2 saturation stable.

The baby girl nursed well the first day, the boy tried, but then got tired. I hand expressed some colostrum and spoon fed it to him. He was alert but small, compared to his sister. He behaved like an IUGR baby. The Balinese midwives also kept vigilant watch over this baby.

Robin would call on the phone and pop in often, to make sure he was improving. It was a team effort.

At 8:00 pm (about 15 hours after birth) I was able to take baby boy off of oxygen and his O2 saturation was 97% on room air! Hallelujah! They are both doing so well. Little by little he was doing better with breastfeeding. A few hours later it became apparent that Radomir, the boy, needed blue light therapy for elevated bilirubin. He was on the bili light, skin-to-skin with his mother, for 12 hours, and his jaundice resolved. When he went off the bili light, his sister, Milanda, then needed 12 hours of photo therapy as well. It was a blessing that Bumi Sehat has a bili blanket, and can look after these babies, who otherwise would have been separated from their mother, and taken off of mother's breast milk, in the hospital.

At one of the postpartum visits, the Mom told me that I taught her ways to breast feed that no one in Russia had ever showed her and she thanked me. She and her babies quickly took to the double football method.

We also found out, after the babies were born, that Olga was a VBAC! I didn't realize that before the birth. I guess her scar was hidden in a fold under her belly. She told me that she went to 27 doctors in Russia and none of them would do a VBAC with her. Like Ibu Robin, I probably would not have accepted her if she had asked to come to The Farm, to have her babies, there were just too many risks. I am glad it all worked out so well for her.

Summing up this Birth...

We midwives have spent time reviewing this twin birth at Bumi Sehat. It was much more dramatic than other twin births we had been the guardians of. This was a VBAC, a twin birth, the 2nd baby slipped out of optimal vertex position to transverse and was born breech! Four midwives from four countries had pushed every boundary that night. We did it for love, and all the right reasons, but we were crazy to do it. We had to do it, because we BELIEVE in Birth and we BELIEVED in Olga and her babies.

Does Your Midwife Support Breastfeeding?

At the beginning of prenatal care you should also find out if your midwife, or doctor, and/or pediatrician really and truly support breastfeeding. In some parts of the world many hospitals, doctors and even midwives promote infant formula, because they get bonuses including money, television sets, gas stoves, even motorbikes, from the infant formula manufacturers, if they encourage bottle feeding, stay away from her. The most important thing about breastfeeding start-up is for the baby and mother not to be separated at the time of birth. The baby must be allowed to stay right up on the mother, skin-to-skin, where he or she can find the breast and initiate breastfeeding within the first ½ hour or 1st hour or so following birth.

Some doctors and midwives work in hospitals that endorse infant formula, because they get cash kick-backs for doing so. It is wise to check the rate of bottle-feeding at the hospital where your Obgyn works. This is easy to do, sit in the lobby and watch the mothers who are discharging to go home with new babies. Are some or all of them holding bottles to their babies' lips? Once the birth is finished, your well meaning Obgyn will have no say about your baby remaining with you, nor will s/he have the power to make sure your baby is not given bottles of infant formula. The Pediatrician, will have dominion over your baby. It is up to you to keep your baby with you, skin to skin, to initiate and maintain breastfeeding in the early hours and days after the birth. Do not even allow the hospital staff to take Baby away for baths. Bathing Baby so soon after birth is not necessary, and being taken away from you will cause trauma. After you go home, after Baby is a week or so old, begin to gently safely bathe him or her in warm water.

Midwives and doctors who take the baby away from the mothers and claim to "help out" by giving the baby milk in a bottle, until the milk comes in, are sabotaging breastfeeding. The infant formula companies know that a high percentage of babies who are given a bottle, even just one bottle of infant formula following birth, will have a very difficult time breastfeeding.

These corporations depend upon midwives, doctors (especially pediatricians), and hospitals to promote infant formula, so that they can increase their business. It is very expensive to bottle-feed a baby. Many couples find themselves tricked into bottle-feeding, and trapped into needing to borrow money constantly, just to feed the baby. For many people, in Indonesia and the Philippines, where I work, the mother or father's salary is not enough to buy the milk needed to bottle feed the baby. Imagine the frustration. Added to the expense of the milk is the cost of medical care for a bottle fed baby. Since breastfed babies are naturally healthier, they go to the doctor much less and nearly never require medicines. The bottle fed baby, on the other hand, is often sick and requires expensive doctor visits and medications much more often.

The best way to be sure your baby breastfeeds is to choose a midwife or birth attendant, and birth-place that will not separate mother from baby at birth. You need a birth attendant who not only believes in breastfeeding, but who helps you to get started and makes sure breastfeeding is easy for both you and your baby, before sending you home to cope on your own.

Research proves that breastfed babies are healthier and more intelligent. In Indonesia and in the Philippine islands, it is national policy to support breastfeeding to protect the coming generation. Don't let a midwife, or doctor, who cares more about promoting infant formula for his or her own profit, trick you into bottle-feeding. It's just not fair to your Baby nor your family. Please, do not be shy, you must protect your own baby by choosing a midwife or doctor who believes in exclusive breastfeeding for the first six months of life. After the first six months, continue to feed baby and introduce age-appropriate foods, one at a time.

The Environmental impact of bottle feeding babies infant formula

First of all, the "milk" produced by corporations for babies, should be called "Artificial Milk" because it in no way resembles human mother's milk, which is the only real healthy option for human babies.

What many families do not know is that bottle feeding babies artificial milk, aka infant formula, actually leads to deforestation, because the "baby milk" companies clear forests and wild lands, to make space to graze cattle. In addition, the off gasses from the waste produced by these cows, who by the way, are NOT being lovingly raised, contributes to the greenhouse effect, a cause of global warming. The packaging (tin and paper and plastic) and transport of infant formula milk greatly contributes to pollution.[9]

Baby formula companies are greatly contributing to the global ecological crisis. They have no respect for our environment, and they profit by hijacking the lives of women, by undermining breastfeeding. Corporations that make and sell baby formula create their market, by setting up mothers to fail at breastfeeding! They do this via advertizing, convincing people that their product is superior to mother's milk.

More evil is the introduction of baby formula, right at the fulcrum of birth. All over the world, doctors and midwives who have taken an oath, to never do harm, accept "gifts" from baby formula corporations. These "gifts" range from new automobiles, motorcycles, television sets, trips abroad, cash, gas stoves, refrigerators, and more. In order to get the "gifts" the doctors, nurses and midwives must addict each baby born in the health facility they work in, to the bottle.

How do they do it? Right at the time of birth, these corrupt healthcare providers immediately clamp and cut the baby's umbilical cord, and send the baby away, to be measured, weighed and separated from mother, undermining First Embrace and breastfeeding start-up. Baby milk corporations even finance the "Baby Room," where the hospital staff (bought off by the corporations) keeps the babies in solitary confinement, feeding them baby formula.

When mothers finally get their babies back in their arms, the babies have suffered profound trauma, and have become conditioned to take the artificial nipples and suck artificial milk from bottles. This habit is hard to overcome. Once a newborn baby has been fed artificial milk aka baby formula, from a bottle, breastfeeding start-up is so much more difficult, and the corporations, like Nestle, Dannon and their partners know this, and they know babies die from the consequences of use of their products. There is a WHO/UNICEF International Code of Marketing that prohibits these unethical practices, but greed prevails. This International Code was adopted to protect mothers,babies and families from unethical and aggressive company practices and to help save the lives of the one and a half million infants who die every year because they are bottl fed.

Mother's Milk, YOUR milk, is one of the Earth's most precious and renewable organic resources.

"Every day, more than 4,000 babies die because they're not breastfed. That's not conjecture, it's UNICEF fact."
~ statement successfully defended before the Advertising Standards Authority by Baby Milk Action

"Some 1.5 million children still die every year because they are inappropriately fed, less than 35% of infants worldwide are exclusively breastfed for the first four months of life, and complementary feeding practices are frequently inappropriate and unsafe."
~ World Health Assembly in May 2001 WHO presented its Global Strategy for Infant and Young Child Feeding

Is My Milk Toxic?

If you are concerned about environmental toxins in your own milk, stay as far away from pollutants, industrial chemicals, and household chemicals as you can. Consider that cows whose milk is in infant formula, are also exposed to pollution, therefore baby formula milk is also contaminated. The benefits of breastfeeding baby, far outweigh any possible ill effects of toxins in mother's milk. A Scientific American article states:

"Although breast milk tends to attract heavy metals and other contaminants due to its high-fat and protein content, some recent research has shown its toxic load to be smaller than that in the air most city dwellers breathe inside their homes"

To make an informed choice about the benefits of Breastfeeding Vs the risks of Infant Formula feeding, see: www.flbreastfeeding.org

Mothers and their families make the decision to breastfeed or bottle feed their baby, based on many sources. Please do not allow corporations who do not care about you, your baby, and our precious planet, to manipulate your decision. The only organic and truly earth friendly, way to feed human babies, is breastfeeding. Run from anyone who tries to convince you otherwise.

A Sad Baby Feeding Story...

"I had a wonderful gentle homebirth, my midwives supported me in everyway and my baby went straight to my breasts and fed, just minutes after she was born. Breastfeeding was going well, until two months latter, someone in my neighborhood mentioned that my daughter was very tiny. She alluded to the fact that she had a niece, who was fed infant formula, who was the same age as my baby, but much fatter. I began to doubt my own milk.

I called my midwives, and they assured me that they were available for a free consult, if I was worried. They asked me how many times per 24 hour day baby wets her diapers, and I said, "More than a dozen." They informed me that this was good news. I did not own a baby scale, but to me she felt like she was getting heavier. My Baby was meeting all her landmarks developmentally. My midwives live 1.5 hours north of me. They offered to come see me. I told them I would come to them. They had come so many times, for postpartum care. I guess I felt shy, to bring them all that distance, just because I was insecure, my baby was perfectly healthy, after all.

Then the same neighbor said, "You should go to this midwife, she is nearby and she can weigh your baby and advise you." I had met with this particular midwife once in early pregnancy, and we did not resonate, so I sought my midwives out, though they practice further away from my town. Anyway, I thought, why not go for a consult to this nearby midwife.

I don't want to mention her name, because I don't want to speak ill of anyone, but this midwife was so harsh. She weighed my baby and scolded me for letting her stay so small, she said I was negligent as a mother. She pinched my breast and milk came, she said, "See how thin your milk is, NOT good. You are starving your baby. You must begin bottle feeding her, immediately. She forced me to buy bottles, artificial nipples and infant formula from her, right then and there. I went home and cried, as I made my baby her first bottle. She drank it, or rather it ran down her throat. As my daughter slept, I cried. I called my midwives and they advised me not to use anymore of the infant formula, but to continue breastfeeding. They emailed me lists of healthy organic foods, which would help me make more milk. I was shattered. I was so insecure that I began to ignore phone calls from them, and I continued to pour the infant formula into my baby. She became ill. I went to the doctor. Her weight was not improving. The doctor encouraged me to keep bottle feeding.

Three more months passed. My baby's weight has hardly gone up at all. She is sick every two to three weeks. When I was exclusively breastfeeding, she was never ill. My milk has dried up. When I try to put her to my breasts, she cries. My midwives came to see me, and they felt so bad. They blamed themselves for not getting in the car, and rushing over to see me, after our first phone call about this. I'm the one who discouraged them. We all feel so terrible. The one who is suffering the most is my baby. I am a single mother, and the cost of this baby formula is painful for me to afford. At night, instead of just giving my baby my breasts to soothe and nourish her. I have to get up and make the bottle. I know I should boil the milk for one hour, to prevent infection from Sakazakii and other bacterias. But I am so tired, and I just mix it up quick, and give her the bottle, to stop my baby's crying. This bottle feeding is a nightmare, I wish I could wake up."

~ **Samantha a mom**

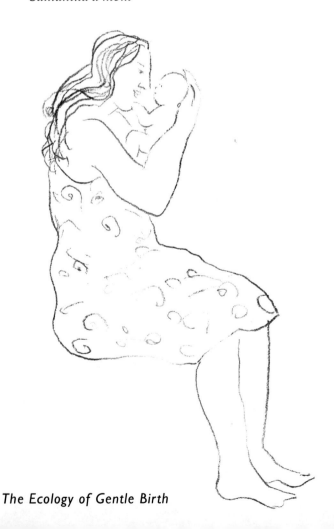

One More thing... before your birth...

If you are blessed to be in a "couple" here is what I would say to you in the last days of your pregnancy: "Take this beautiful couple on a date." Yup, that's right, a proper date, with candle light, exchange little gifts, flirt, feed each other, dance, enjoy and if it feels right ... make love.

"Why a date?" you may ask. Because once this baby is born, the relationship you are in now will change so much, that you really become a different couple. So, it's really a goodbye date. "Goodbye," to the couple you have been and, "Welcome," to the couple you will be, as parents. This date will be sweet, and you may shed some tears. This is the couple who invited this Baby to Earth. The arrival of Baby is both a birth and a rebirth. Birth of a Baby, and a rebirth of the parents, anew. Rebirth is predicated by a kind of death. Properly give this couple a send off, place those precious memories on a special shelf in your hearts. Then, from time to time, take that couple down, and visit with them. They will strengthen and guide your love when you most need it. Keep them close in your hearts, but accept that you are about to change utterly and astonishingly.

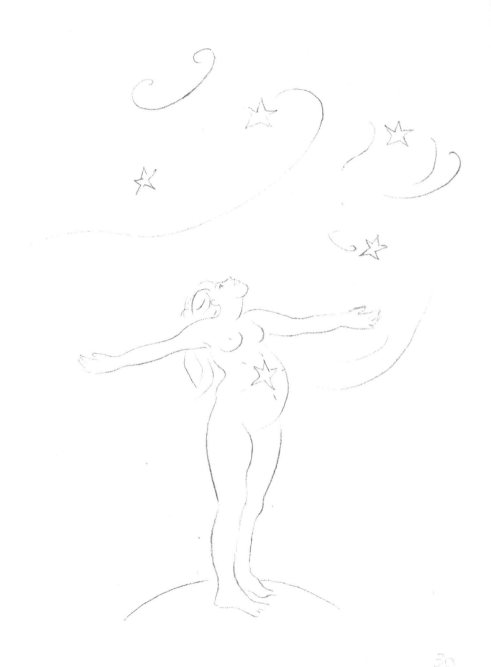

Birth the Miracle

...Ready or not, Baby is arriving!

Just so you know... Today about 353,000 women will give birth. Your contractions join with theirs, to bring miracle babies to Earth... may all be blessed.

Have I begun Labor?

First you will notice signs of labor beginning. Perhaps your mucus plug will come out, this is sometimes called the "bloody show" because of the pink tinge or red seen in the mucous (if it's clear or yellowish mucous, not pink or a bit blood stained, it's not the real thing, YET.) Not all mothers notice a bloody show. If you do, consider it like a letter from the baby saying:

> *"I'm fixing to begin labor with you, within the next 24 or 48 hours or so. Get some extra rest mom. Load up on carbohydrates and comfort foods, because we are going to need some energy. If you have anything you wished to do, before my arrival, now is the time, because I plan to capture ALL of your attention. I love you."*
>
> *~ Baby*

If you have been having Braxton Hicks contractions, your body has been warming up nicely for labor. If you have been letting go, really leaning into the sensation of the Braxton-Hicks contractions, preparing yourself physically and spiritually for the full-blown miracle, then you still really have no idea what it's all about. Even after four births, I was amazed at the intensity of labor when it really got going, for my fifth time! This is something truly impossible to articulate. Amazing and challenging as it is, there is a part of you, perhaps deep in each of your cells, which once labor has begun, says; "Yes, I KNOW what this is." Perhaps we "know" because labor contractions feel utterly natural, and as women, we were made to birth our babies.

I have begun labor many ways. The first time I gave birth, my water broke (amniotic fluid released), and contractions began. Four and a half hours later I was holding my first baby! My next experience of childbirth began with the slow onset of regular contractions. Labor with my third baby began with strong regular contractions, five minutes apart. Because of my reputation for giving birth quickly, my midwife immediately drove for two hours, from the east side of Maui, drinking strong Earl Grey tea, along the way. I was worried that she would not make it, as my contractions increased in intensity and were soon three minutes apart. When Midwife arrived, she hugged me and listened to my baby's heartbeat. She went to the kitchen to make me some herbal tea, and when she came back to my bedside, I had fallen asleep! She of course could not sleep, and sat up all night, chatting with an old friend of mine who was visiting from Iowa. My labor had completely stopped, and did not resume, until more than a week later. That old friend from Iowa never forgot meeting my midwife. Years latter, when she died, he helped support her son through college. I had been so shy, having woken my midwife and gotten her to drive so far, at such an hour. How happy I was, when the story unfolded, and I realized that my baby had a plan, which none of us would see, for many years to come.

Practice labor is not uncommon. I don't call it "false labor" because those contractions feel REAL, and they do help bring the baby, they count! Don't be shy about calling your midwife if you think you've begun labor. She or he is accustomed to "test runs," so don't be embarrassed if you have one or two, or more. Like I said earlier, I believe that there is no such thing as false labor. Every contraction adds up and contributes to bringing the baby Earth-side.

Vivi had her first baby breech, naturally and gently at the Bumi Sehat Birth home. Five years later, as she was expecting her second baby, having a head-down baby felt very odd to her. For the last two and ½ weeks of her pregnancy, she thought she was in true labor many times. Her Husband would borrow a car and bring her to the midwives at the birth center. Usually within an hour of arriving, in what seemed to be real labor, Vivi would fall asleep, and wake up in the morning, refreshed and confused that labor had begun and then stopped.

Finally the midwives invited Vivi to have an ultrasound scan with them. During the scan it was found that Vivi's baby's placenta was low-lying, quite low. This is called a "marginal placena." It did not cover the cervix nor prevent the baby's head from descending down into the pelvis. The midwives reassured Vivi, that it was OK. Vivi in tears shared that she had been to a doctor in early pregnancy. He told her she would definitely need a cesarean, due to a low-lying placenta. This frightened her so much, and she was afraid to even tell her midwives, afraid they would not help her with her birth, if they knew. Once this fear was out in the open, and Vivi had a good cry, she went home, had a good night's sleep, and came back in strong real labor. Three hours later, Vivi's daughter was gently born, just as she had dreamed, into the hands of her trusted midwives. There were not complications at all.

What IF my water breaks?

Sometimes a pregnant mother feels wetness in her underpants, only to find it is her juicy pregnancy fluids, or pee has leaked. If your feel a gush or leak of body temperature, fluid, that does not smell like urine, you water or amniotic fluid may have released. Sometimes it has little white flecks of vernix, the creamy coating of the baby's skin. Your midwife or doctor can use litmus paper to determine if your baby's waters have released.

If this happens, pay close attention to hygiene. No tub baths. If you are planning a water birth your midwife will wish for you to wait to get into the tub, until you are in active labor and have dilated 5 centimeters or more. You may take showers. Once your amniotic fluid has released, or is leaking, you should not make love. Nothing that is not absolutely sterile should enter your vagina. When using the toilet always wipe from front to back, so as not to introduce bacteria into your vagina. This is good hygiene always, but especially important if your waters have released, because now the baby is no longer sealed safely away from bacteria.

With my last baby, Wayan Hanoman, my water released just before sunrise and nothing happened, until the sunset on that day. If your water releases, let your midwife know. Follow careful hygiene, be sure to wipe from front to back when using toilet. Showers are fine if your amniotic fluids have released, but baths are not. No love making after waters have released. You must take these simple precautions to make sure bacteria does not get into your uterus and affect Baby.

Many women feel a burst of energy. Before one of my births I woke up in the morning and vomited. Then I felt energized. I ate, cleaned my house, top to bottom and then rested. I even finished sewing my baby's quilt. That night labor began.

I had a good cry, an absolute "give up" just about 1 ½ hours before the first signs of labor began, four out of five times.

There is a tingle in the air, which enlivens everyone around, when a woman is in labor. Many midwives and obstetricians have described it as "Psychedelic." I believe that we can feel the Angels coming to help.

If you see blood, call your midwife, straight away. Together you can determine how much blood, and why. Also, if your waters break, try to sop it up with a white towel, so you can see if it is clear or not. If the amniotic fluid has a yellow or green tinge to it, tell your midwife or doctor immediately, as it could indicate that the baby has passed meconium, which is newborn poop. Sometimes it means the baby is mature and ready for birth, sometimes, if it is thick meconium, like pea soup, it tells the midwife that the baby had some distress, and that she must pay special attention to monitoring this wee one during your labor. If your waters have released, and this is not your first baby, you should go straight away to the birth clinic, hospital where you plan to birth. If you are having a home birth, call the midwife to let her know. She will want arrive by your side quite soon. After the waters have released, labor usually beings quite spontaneously, if not right away, within a few hours. If it does not, you midwife will have some tricks-or-the-trade, to help encourage labor to earnestly begin.

Deborah's Stair Steps of Labor

Something I tell pregnant women the last part of their pregnancy, to help them prepare for labor:

When the contractions feel strong, if you breathe through them, and try to relax and let the endorphins flow, usually after a few contractions, you can integrate them better, and it does not seem so intense.

Then as labor progresses, and the contractions become more intense again, going up to a new level, if you can remember that it did that before, and you DID learn how to integrate it, you handled it just fine. With this new intensity, you can do that again. You can think of it like stair steps, it goes up to a new level, then it plateaus for a while.

When the next stair step rises, the more you have faith in your capacity to cope, the smoother it will go. Have Faith that your body knows what it's doing. Stay out of labor's way, let your body do it. Sometimes you just have to ride the wave, surrender to the force. When you BELIEVE in yourself, it all unfolds perfectly.

Some women get meditative in their surrender to the strength and intensity of the contractions. It's almost like self-hypnosis, when you surrender, the pain is there, but it feels like less.

Even though the contractions grow stronger, it's not hurting as much as it did in early labor, because you are handling it and surrendering better and better.

Deborah Flowers
Farm Midwife

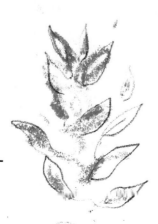

Who Can Accompany Me?

*"Women do better in childbirth in a warm, safe place,
where they do not feel watched or judged, with the help of
a mother or trusted mother-figure to help them."*

~ Dr. Michel Odent

It is every woman's right to choose WHERE, with WHO and HOW
she wants to labor and birth her baby. Of course, IF there are overrid-
ing risks to you or your baby, this will influence your choice of birth
location and attendants.

Before your baby is due to be born, make sure your midwife will
allow your husband or partner, and/or your doula, mother, sister, or
dear friend, or an aunt, whoever you trust, to be with you as a support
person through labor and delivery of your baby. You should never be
forced to be alone, without the people you love beside you, supporting you. With your doula and your mother or sister or dear friend rub-
bing your back, labor will be shorter. One special look and touch from
your partner, will give you courage. Labor is hard work, and yet you
must relax to allow your body to do her job of bringing the baby earth-
side. For this kind of work, you need loving support, from people who
BELIEVE in you, and who trust birth. Also, you must let anyone you
have invited to your birth know that if an emergency arises, or if you
simply feel you have changed your mind about who you need beside
you, you may ask them to leave. Each person in your birth-team must
be completely open to what MotherBaby need. Birth is not a specta-
tor sport. So it is best not to invite people to just come watch. Only
include helpers who have a role and who you feel 100% comfortable
with. Some midwives feel that for each "extra" or "not needed" person
at the birth, labor could be prolonged by an extra hour. I am not sure
about this, for it is so individual and of course culture plays a role.
Each mother for each baby must be empowered to choose who will
be supporting her during labor and birth. We are after all mammalian
creatures, and we need to be free to move and find the right space
physically, mentally, spiritually and socially, to give birth. We need to
feel free to howl, to poop, and to laugh while crying. We need to nest,
and go outside in the air and feel the grass between our toes. We need
support and privacy, all at once.

Doulas ~ Weaving the Circle of Support

"If a woman doesn't look like a goddess during labor, then someone isn't treating her right."

~ Ina May Gaskin

Before Doctors or formally trained midwives, even before there were hospitals or clinics, or homes as we know them today, women helped and supported women through pregnancy, childbirth and postpartum. Women created a circle of support for the childbearing mother and her family. Today the Doula is re-weaving this ancient circle of support, bringing female companionship back to the time-honored tradition of women supporting women during childbirth.

Doula is the Greek word that means, "one who mothers or serves the mother." Being a doula is the loving art of mothering the new mother. Traditionally women were cared for in the loving arms of mothers from their own families and tribes, as they made the miraculous and sometimes challenging journey, of bringing a baby to earth. Doula, like midwife, but with different roles, are the most time-honored ancient occupations.

Today Doulas bring expertise in comfort techniques for pregnancy, labor and birth. They are not medically trained, so they are not a replacement for your midwife or doctor. If you are blessed to have a life partner, they are not meant to replace him/her. They are purely there to support you, and your healthy journey into motherhood. Your doula will help you form a birth vision. Your doula will rub your back, yes… and she will do so much more. She will even teach your partner how to best comfort you. She will advocate for you and believe in you. In fact, because women who have doulas have much lower rates of cesarean, some insurance companies will pay a doula to come with you to the hospital. This is because it saves the insurance company money!

In the U.S two states have passed legislation for Doula coverage and more states and countries are considering Doulas to improve childbirth outcomes, reduce costs, increase satisfaction and long term positive birth memories.

Normally you will meet your doula during pregnancy. She will help you prepare spiritually and mentally for the birth ahead. There are also doulas who guide and care for you in the postpartum period. I highly recommend both pregnancy/birth doulas and postpartum doulas. Your doula will work closely with your midwife and/or doctor. She has a wealth of knowledge about pregnancy, birth, postpartum and breastfeeding. She will not just answer your questions, she will guide you to discover your own inner knowing. You don't need to look for your inner knowing, your authentic self, it's always been there. Unfolding as a mother will help you get in touch with your awake and wonderful inner knowing.

The World Health Organization document, The prevention and elimination of disrespect and abuse during facility-based childbirth, states: "Greater action is needed to support changes in provider behavior, clinical environments and health systems to ensure that all women have access to respectful, competent and caring maternity health care services. This can include (but is not limited to) social support through a companion of choice."

Understanding the unique role and scope of practice of Doulas as well as the benefits and cost savings will encourage families to arrange for Doula care, Today's midwives are inspired to work in collaboration with Doulas, to enhance quality compassionate care.

Midwives face many challenges balancing professionalism, responsibilities of the job, the desire to give each laboring/birthing mother continuous care, in both out-of-hospital & hospital birth settings. I have found that even while practicing midwifery in high risk, low resource environments, like Indonesia after earthquakes, tsunamis and terrorist bombings, Philippines following typhoons, optimal MotherBaby care is best achieved by collaborating with Doulas.

While not interfering the healthcare providers' practice, Doulas offer a solution that makes space for midwives and doctors to improve their performance at birth, just by lowering the birthing mothers stress, thereby reducing the strain on midwives and collaborating Obgyns.

I firmly believe: Doulas are here to stay. Women love them. By forging progressive partnerships, BirthKeepers and families may enter into a more enlightened age of optimal, respectful MotherBaby care, highlighted by improved outcomes and happier, more satisfied mothers.

"I believe that in order to have natural childbirth in any hospital in New York City, you must have your doula with you."

~ Eden Fromberg, Doctor of Obstetrical Medicine

"Too many women labor alone, and in the last 50 years male partners are replacing female companions. Growing data demonstrates the benefits of returning to continuous female companionship, including Doulas, during labor, birth and postpartum. A Doula is trained to provide emotional and physical comfort and care for laboring/ birthing mothers. For partners and family members, the Doula adds stability and becomes a pillar for coping. Data strongly states that, a Doula must not be a part of the hospital system, but rather a beneficial adjunct to Midwife-to-Mother care. The Cochrane reviews states that "Continuous support during labour should be the norm, rather than the exception... policy makers should consider including doulas as a covered benefit for all women."

~ Debra Pascali-Bonaro, acclaimed filmmaker of "Orgasmic Birth," Mother, Grandmother and Doula

Labor and Birth Positions...

Laying on one's back is most often not the most powerful or efficient and comfortable way to have a baby. Here are some ideas of how you may wish to labor and birth your baby. Women around the world give birth in many different positions. It is believed to be easier to be assisted by gravity, by pushing the baby downward, instead of upward. This makes sense, however, some mothers just want to lay down! I gave birth five times, and each time in a different position. In fact I often wonder if my husband really caught our son, Hanoman, or if he bungee bounced out of me to the floor! I was standing up with my arms thrown around Wil's neck when our 5th child arrived, with a slippery gush! Our son still jokes and says, "Dad, did you drop me?"

Experiment in labor, move your body to find positions most comfortable for you. Even in our day and age, all over the world, women are forced to give birth on high obstetrical tables, with their feet in stirrups. This position goes against our mammalian maternal instinct, to birth close to our Earth Mother. It is cruel, and must be changed. Even in this day and age, Doulas in Los Angeles California tell me that have seen women brought to hospital from the prison, and chained to the Obstetrical table, in stirrups. Personally, I am on a campaign to eliminate the obstetrical table and stirrups from birth rooms all over the planet! It is a basic human right, to be supported to give birth in any position that comforts you. If dogs were forced to give birth in the ways I have seen women forced birth in, in hospitals all over the planet, there would be a public outcry against it.

What about Labor?

YES, labor and childbirth are challenging. You will need courage to face this life passage. Many mothers have benefitted from acknowledging their fears and clearing the way spiritually and mentally to gentle birth. Remember, you are a creature, and your body knows how to birth, just as the she wolves and the bears know how.

Positive & Strengthening Thoughts ~ Please add your own to this list....

- My Baby is growing to the perfect size for my body to birth naturally.
- My Baby is in the perfect position to birth smoothly.
- My pelvis is strong, open & flexible, she moves to allow my Baby through.
- I am responsible for MY Birth MY Baby.
- I now choose to have a loving, gentle natural birth.
- Through my contractions I will find strength.
- Through Birth I will find healing.
- My Baby is safe and instinctively knows all is well.
- Instinctively, I know exactly what to do to bring my Baby into this world.
- I trust that my midwives care and are skilled to assist me in this miracle.
- My Birth Support Team has my back, and my front, side and middle.
- I am supported by Mother Earth, Father Sky gives me wings and imagination.
- Just as the flower opens to greet the morning sun, my cervix opens fully.
- I stay centered and balanced in my labor.
- I welcome and surrender to each contraction as I bring my Baby to Earth.
- I call upon the wisdom of birthing women through all time to guide & help.
- I feel the song of All Mothers' strength in childbirth. I sing it now!
- I know the dance of women birthing. I dance it now!
- I bring my Baby out, into the light.
- I am a creature, a daughter of the Earth Mother, who is holding me in her protective arms, while Father Time guides me.
- I celebrate the power of my partnership with my Divine Creator in birthing this Baby.

Affirmations...

- *I have ample courage to face these amazing changes in my life.*
- *Baby... thank you for kicking, and letting me know just how ALIVE we are together.*
- *Baby... I trust that you are with me, designing a perfect birth plan for both of us.*

> "There is a secret in our culture and it is not that birth is painful but that women are strong."
>
> ~ Laura Stavoe

Gentle Birth.... Respectful Care

> "The parallels between making love and giving birth are clear, not only in terms of passion and love, but also because we need essentially the same conditions for both experiences: privacy and safety. "
>
> ~ Sarah Buckley

Doctor and Home/Lotus Birth mOM

Gentle birth means that during the process of labor and birth the MotherBaby are being respected and supported and loved by her family members as well her midwives and or doctor and nurses. In many parts of our planet we still have skilled Dukun Bayi (Indonesian traditional birth helpers) also known as Hilots (in the Philippines), Traditional Birth Attendants who help women at the time of birth and postpartum. They are often gifted with experience and wisdom. Today we bring together the wisdom of these grandmothers, along with the sisterly tenderness of our Doulas, the motherly medical skills of our midwives or doctors, may they work in concert to BELIEVE in each woman and support her journey into Motherhood.

In gentle birth the woman may choose her birth location, be it hospital, birth clinic, midwifery practice, or home. She may also choose what position she wishes to birth in, laying, squatting, side lying, semi-sitting, all fours, standing, etc…

No one must harm your body or spirit. I have witnessed insults and even slaps and punches thrown at laboring mothers in hospitals. Obstetrical violence has been forced upon women in many countries, at the hands of cruel misguided birth attendants. It is time to break the silence.

The age of ignorance is ending. Midwives, doulas, nurses and doctors today are trained to be kind, skilled, loving and supportive during labor and birth. An expectant mother may expect to be treated with kindness and respect.

Some examples of non-respectful childbirth practices:

- Forcing a laboring mother to be up on a high Ob table for her birth goes against our mammalian instinct to stay close to the Mother Earth while birthing, it is cruel. The high OB tables can be narrow and the mother perceives a danger for her baby, after the birth. The hospitals remove the baby from the mother's arms, quickly, afraid she will drop her baby, from a table not designed for mother-baby bonding. They were designed for the comfort of doctors "delivering" babies, forgetting that actually the mothers deliver their babies. The OB table is not at all practical or kind for Mothers and Babies.

- A laboring and birthing mother should be encouraged to move, walk and dance, choosing her own positions. Confining her to a bed for labor, or and OB table, often hooked up to a fetal monitor, is cruel and prolongs labor.

- Unless absolutely needed for the safety of the baby, continuous fetal monitoring during labor has been shown not to improve outcomes. It forces the mother to stay still in a bed during labor, and impedes progress.

- Ignoring a laboring and birthing mother's need for privacy, loving support, and comfort measures, like massage, water therapy, continuous care from a loving family member and/or a doula, is uncompassionate.

- Withholding food and fluids is disrespectful and not necessary unless the mother is preparing for a cesarean birth. Labor is hard work, and mothers need their fuel, food and fluids.

- Putting a woman's labor on a progress time-line, forcing her to conform to a prescribed time when her birth "should" take place, is also cruel. This all to often can lead to a unnecessary cesarean birth, compounding trauma.

- Pushing violently on the fundus (belly of the pregnant mom) is not good medicine. It may dangerous and not at all gentle.

- Episiotomies, cutting the vaginal opening to make it bigger for childbirth is almost never necessary, and it is not recommended in the International standards for Normal Childbirth.

- Separating the mother from her family during labor and birth, forcing her to make this exceptional life passage surrounded by strangers, is cruel.

- Immediate (or quite fast ie severing the cord before it truly stops pulsing) clamping and cutting of the Baby's umbilical cord, is terrible. It is a practice that harms babies.

- Separating the MotherBabyPlacenta trinity causes trauma, it must not be done. Even if a baby needs to be resuscitated at birth, this can be done right beside the mother, or even between her legs. (there are now infant resuscitation tables that roll right up to the mother, so babies cords may stay intact during resuscitation. Babies survive better if they can feel mother is right there, touching the baby calling for him or her, during the neonatal resuscitation. Babies who are still connected to the unclamped umbilical cord during neonatal resuscitation, are getting oxygen, iron, nutrients and stem cell rich blood from the placenta via the cord, this supports life and the success of Neonatal Resuscitation.

- Manufacturing the need for cesarean birth, when it is not truly necessary causes trauma and hardship for the mother, baby and family. When unnecessary cesareans are being done, the surgeons and operating rooms, are less available when a true emergency arises, delaying care for mothers and babies in verifiable need.

Childbirth works best, if we leave our thinking brain behind, and allow our most basic mammalian instincts to take over, and lead us through the experience. If the mother is put in a situation that shames, isolates or frightens her, labor will be impaired and a cascade of interventions will ensue. Mammals in their natural habitat do not give birth when disturbed. People are mammals. The survival mechanism: fight or flight, sabotages our innate ability to bring babies Earth-side, without interventions or complications.

> *"Let's say you want some advice that might help you give birth, wherever that might be. My shortest answer is: let your monkey do it."*
>
> *~ Ina May Gaskin*

Pushing... aka 2nd Stage

> *"Pushing was like swimming under water—when you want to come up for air you can usually stay just a little longer. So when I'd feel like giving up during a push, I'd say to myself, "Push a little harder, this may be the one!"*
>
> *~ Deborah Flowers*

The ebbs and flows, challenges and triumphs of labor will at some point give way, and you will feel a change. This change may well mean you are fully dilated to 10 centimeters and your baby is nice and low presenting upon your perineum. This means you are ready to push. You may not have a choice, because for some women the fetal ejection reflex is so compelling a feeling that you MUST push. Some mothers feel like they are pooping a watermelon! Don't worry, you yoni was designed to stretch, your baby's head is molding to fit perfectly... YOU GOT THIS.

Some laboring mothers may feel the urge to push, before their cervix is fully dilated. Waiting until this feeling passes can be super challenging. Breathe, (as if that will help) actually it helps the baby stay oxygenated and more comfortable. Move, change positions, pee if you can, because a full bladder can make you feel a lot of pressure down below, on your perineum. Ask your birth companions, family and/or doula, to massage your back and legs. Hold on, if you can dilate to 7 or 8 centimeters, you will dilate to 10. If you are planning a WaterBirth, and you tub is ready, getting in the water can give you so much relief that the urge to push, before full dilation can be handled better.

Some mothers, especially those who are not having a first baby, may wish not to consciously push, but to allow their baby to emerge, pushed only by the force of the contractions of hr uterus. During 2nd stage, you and your midwives will know if this is the best way for you and your baby.

Some mothers, like me, can feel like they are at the end of their strength, only to find that baby is very low and the cervix is full dilated. They may push! Wow, that pushing feels like, "I am amazing, labor is not doing me, I am pushing, I am fierce and strong and on top of this. YES, I can birth this Baby! I found pushing was less painful that not pushing. It was a triumph to push my baby into the light.

> "At the moment of birth, there is a rare and brief glimpse of the connection between this world and another, of before and after, of mortal and immortal, of spiritual and physical, of known and unknown." ~ **Ida Darragh**

> "You're braver than you believe. Stronger than you seem. And smarter than you think."
>
> ~ **Christopher Robin in Pooh's Grand Adventure**

The Necessary Question of Infants' Human Rights at Birth...

Are there Vampires in the Birth Rooms? (*from Ibu Robin's book: Placenta the Forgotten Chakra*)

Parents, grandparents, aunts, uncles, siblings, families, midwives, doulas, doctors, nurses, hospital administrators and legislators... we are BirthKeepers. It is our responsibility to ask the next question concerning human rights in childbirth. As BirthKeepers, it is we who are given the sacred responsibility to protect the mothers and our incoming humans, the newborns, at birth and as they grow, for they are the future EarthKeepers.

My question:

Are we allowing our health providers to rob our babies of their full potential of health, intelligence, immunity and longevity, at birth?

According to the American Red Cross, blood donors must be in good health, at least 17 years old in most States and weigh at least 110 lbs (50 kg).[10] In Germany, children under the age of 18 are not eligible to donate blood. Blood donations are generally no more than 500 ml, which is 1/10th of the average adult blood volume. Clearly newborn babies do not fit these criteria for donating blood.

At the time of birth up to ⅓ of each baby's blood supply is traveling from the placenta via the umbilical cord to the baby. Calling this blood "cord blood" is doublespeak; intentionally ambiguous language meant to fool parents into misunderstanding. The fact is, the blood present in the umbilical cord at the time of birth is truly the BABY'S blood.

All over the world, in nearly every single medical institution where babies are born, newborns (usually weighing only between 2 and 5 kilos (4.4 to 11 lbs) are being denied up to ⅓ of their blood volume. This happens when the umbilical cord is immediately clamped and cut, by the doctor or midwife, moments after the baby is born. Parents are encouraged to donate their baby's "cord" blood, which in actuality is the baby's blood. Although it may be a generous gift for someone who needs a transfusion, this precious blood supply is meant for the baby and should not be given away or sold.

At the moment of birth, newborn infants have a blood volume of approximately 78 ml/kg, which means about 273 ml, at an average weight of 3.5 kg. This is the diminished amount of blood that almost all newborns are left with when their umbilical cords are immediately clamped and cut.

Research has shown that when umbilical cord clamping is delayed for 5 minutes, a newborn's blood volume increases by 61% to 126 ml/kg, for an average total of 441 ml. This placental transfusion amounts to 168 ml for an average 3.5 kg (7.7 lb.) infant. One-quarter of this transfusion occurs in the first 15 seconds, and one-half within 60 seconds of birth.

My question:
Is taking ⅓ of a mammal's blood supply harmful?

It's unconscionable that it's even legal for hospital protocols and practices to harm newborns by robbing them at birth of so much of their blood. I have reviewed the extensive research and the evidence, and found absolutely NO benefits for newborn babies when their umbilical cords are immediately clamped and cut at the time of birth. In fact, the studies prove this to be a harmful practice.

No parent would sign a waiver (often presented in fine print, as part of a long informed consent given to mother when she arrives at a hospital in labor) giving away ⅓, or any amount, of their baby's blood. Yet, thousands of times, every day and night, parents are deluded into giving away a significant part of their baby's precious blood supply! The majority of parents in the world are not even asked if the baby's umbilical cord may be immediately severed.

I am quite sure that if I were to remove ⅓ of even one adult patient's blood without his or her consent, it would be considered a crime. There would be media outcry against me and I would be prosecuted. How then is it possible that people tolerate the same unfair treatment of human neonates?

A mountain of research shows that by simply delaying the clamping and cutting of babies' umbilical cords, our newborn children suffer less trauma, fewer inner cranial hemorrhages and have higher stores of iron at 4 months of age, and even up to 8 months after birth.[11, 12, 13] The nutrients, oxygen and stem cells present in the blood transfused into babies by the placenta, when cord severance is delayed, ensures that the body's tissues and organs are properly vitalized, supplied with energy and nourished. This translates into improved health, heightened immunity, increased intelligence and potential longevity.

In addition, keeping the umbilical cord intact for some time following birth means that the baby may remain skin to skin with mother. This eliminates or greatly reduces the potential for birth trauma. Research has proven that babies born without trauma enjoy an intact capacity to love and trust. (Michel Odent OBGYN "The Scientification of Love," see entire book)

The simple, natural, common-sense practice of giving the placenta time to do its job, of delivering to the baby his or her full blood supply, has been criticized and NOT implemented by the very doctors and hospitals who have taken an oath, to "Never Do Harm."

The imposed medical habit of immediately clamping and cutting babies' umbilical cords has not been with us so long (just over 200 years) and yet, in the minds of many healthcare providers, it is erroneously considered "normal" and "necessary." Clearly the research proves it is not necessary, nor is it evidenced based practice.

> *"Another thing very injurious to the child, is the tying and cutting of the navel string too soon; which should always be left till the child has not only repeatedly breathed but till all pulsation in the cord ceases. As otherwise the child is much weaker than it ought to be, a portion of the blood being left in the placenta, which ought to have been in the child."*
>
> *~ Erasmus Darwin, Zoonomia, 1801*

My question:

Why do some babies who have had their cords immediately clamped and cut need phototherapy for pathological jaundice?

The habitual practice of immediate umbilical cord clamping and cutting began in the 1960s when an unproven hypothesis arose among physicians, in which they postulated that immediate cord severance would prevent jaundice. Research has proven that there is no greater risk of pathological jaundice for newborns whose cord clamping and cutting is delayed.[14] Research, conducted by Ola Andersson, consultant in neonatology, Lena Hellström-Westas, professor of perinatal medicine, Dan Andersson, head of departments of paediatrics, obstetrics and gynaecology, Magnus Domellöf, associate professor, head of paediatrics, and featured in the British Medical Journal, states: "There were no significant differences between (immediate cord cut and delayed cord cut: mine) groups in postnatal respiratory symptoms, polycythaemia, or hyperbilirubinaemia requiring phototherapy."

Another theory was that early cord clamping would prevent Polycythemia (too much hemoglobin) or hyperviscocity (blood that is too thick.) Some research does show an increased concentration of hemoglobin in the delayed cord clamping group, but it has not harmed babies, nor is it a significant argument for immediate cord severance. Many of the arguments against universally adopting delayed cord clamping and cutting into overall birth protocols are addressed in an article 'Common Objections to Delayed Cord Clamping' by the pediatric physician Mark Sloan M.D. In his summary Dr. Sloan states: "Delayed cord clamping promotes a healthy neonatal cardiopulmonary transition, prevents iron deficiency at a critical time in brain development, provides the newborn with a rich supply of stem cells, and helps sick neonates achieve better outcomes—all with little apparent risk to mother or baby. **The evidence of benefit from DCC is so compelling that the burden of proof must now lie with those who wish to continue the practice of immediate clamping, rather than with those who prefer—as nature intended—to wait."** *(bold type added by Dr. Sloan)*

My questions:

- *What are the Babies' human rights?*

- *Is the practice and protocol of immediate umbilical cord severance harming our children?*

- *Is early umbilical cord severance causing newborn anemia, making babies less alert and thereby sabotaging breastfeeding and bonding?*

- *Is it impairing our children's birthright to their full potential of health and intelligence?*

At this junction of herstory and history, many BirthKeepers are asking these very questions. ,

When immediate umbilical cord clamping and cutting was introduced, it was never questioned. NO research was conducted to determine if it was a safe practice. It was just done for convenience. Doctors, nurses and midwives began to follow the trend, herded like sheep against the fear of asking the next question. Later, they justified it with an erroneous myth about delayed cord severance causing jaundice.

Research proves that immediate or early umbilical cord severance is detrimental to our newborn children, but few healthcare providers seem alarmed. Are we hypnotized? Why are we trusting medical professionals who, in some instances profit from denying our offspring their very blood? Stealing blood is what vampires do.

My question:

Is profit a motivator in the continuation of a practice that research and good sense clearly demonstrates endangers the physical, mental and emotional health of our children?

Stem cells are valuable, blood is valuable, and hospitals sell babies' blood for transfusions and for research and other uses, including transfusion.[18] A simple Google search on "cord blood" demonstrates how many businesses there are surrounding this capital rich issue. Once again I wish to say: "There is no such thing as cord blood, it is the baby's blood." Many parents are asked to donate their baby's (cord blood) to science or to help others. Did you know umbilical cords are marketed for transplants? Placentas have also been sold to cosmetic companies to be used in beauty supplies, though this is now much less common.

The question of cord blood banking arises. First of all, remember that it is actually baby's blood, not cord blood. That said, there are two directions parents are encouraged to choose from: banking their baby's stem-cell-rich blood for donation (presumably to help someone in the future), an altruistic idea; or, banking baby's blood for future personal use (autologous), should the child develop a disease perhaps treatable by blood transfusion. The most touted of the presumably treatable diseases is leukemia. The probability that a person in the course of his or her life will ever need a stem cell transplant (whether from umbilical cord blood or bone marrow) has been estimated by the University Hospital in Heidelberg at 0.06% to 0.46%, depending on age. Correspondingly low, the probability that one's own cord blood would be used in a transplant is between 1: 1400 and 1: 200,000.[19] The technology to properly store this baby blood is still not adequate to insure that the blood will be useable in the future. Parents are driven by fear and love for their baby to pay between 1,500 and 2,000 euros or more for the initial "harvesting" of their baby's blood at birth. Storage programs, for between ten and twenty-five years cost between 90 and 120 euros per year. Parents are asked to gamble that technology will advance enough to make their investment useful, should the worst case scenario for their child's health arise. It must be said out loud and precisely: YOUR BABY NEEDS THAT BLOOD AND STEM CELL INFUSION, WITH ALL ITS BENEFITS, AT THE TIME OF BIRTH, AS NATURE INTENDED IT. With that in mind, there is a third option for parents who are convinced of the need for blood banking: to harvest the baby's blood for collection and storage AFTER delaying the clamping and cutting of baby's umbilical cord, allowing for some of the essential transfusion to take place at the time of birth.

In some countries (especially in the USA), fear of litigation has been used to justify early cord cutting. In 1995, the American Academy of Obstetricians and Gynecologists (ACOG) released an Educational Bulletin (#216) recommending immediate cord clamping in order to obtain cord blood for blood gas studies in case of a future lawsuit. They did this because deviations in blood gas values at birth can reflect asphyxia, or lack of. Lack of asphyxia at birth is viewed as proof in a court of law that a baby was healthy at birth. In other words, ACOG made the recommendation to protect its member doctors, not the babies.

Following an unpublished letter sent to ACOG by Dr. Morley, ACOG withdrew this Educational Bulletin in the February 2002 issue of Obstetrics and Gynecology (the ACOG journal.)[20] This action released them of liability resulting from their previous bulletin #216 of 1995. Parents and all BirthKeepers must ask: WHY, if ACOG has withdrawn its erroneous instruction to doctors to immediately clamp and cut babies' umbilical cords, is it still universally and dangerously practiced?

Midwives and doctors who propose and support the healthy process of placental transfusion at birth by delaying umbilical cord clamping and cutting are criticized and charged with the burden of proving that letting Mother Nature and Father Time take their course at the time of birth is safe! Thinking medical professionals and caring parents and grandparents have concluded that OBGYNs and midwives who insist on routine, immediate umbilical cord cutting are simply protecting their right to practice with impatience, and what they deem 'efficiency,' with no regard for the rights of the baby, who cannot protest.

At Bumi Sehat in Indonesia and the Philippines, we have received nearly 7,000 babies safely into the world, in high-risk, low resource settings, including disaster zones where the patients are homeless, hungry and lack adequate drinking water. All of these babies enjoyed delayed umbilical cord clamping and cutting. Normally we wait 3 hours before doing anything with babies' umbilical cords, and many parents choose keeping the cord and placenta connected to the baby until the cord naturally dries and falls away (Full Lotus Birth.) Both of my grandsons enjoyed this non-violent practice. By waiting for some time, even hours, before performing the cord care, weighing and measuring of baby etc., we insure that the Mother may breastfeed her baby unimpeded by unnecessary interventions and devices (e.g. the cord clamp; which is uncomfortable for baby and mother when the two are skin to skin, having their first breastfeeding and bonding experiences). This opens the way for optimal breastfeeding start-up conditions.

At Bumi Sehat we have experienced NO ill effects to babies from delaying umbilical cord clamping and cutting. In a comparative study looking at the outcomes of 30 babies born of anemic mothers at Bumi Sehat receiving greatly delayed cord severance compared with 30 babies born of anemic mothers born in a local hospital with immediate cord severance, there was NO increased rate of jaundice in the Bumi Sehat babies, and they enjoyed higher hemoglobin levels.[21]

At Bumi Sehat the MotherBabies enjoy a breastfeeding rate of 100% upon discharge from all three of our childbirth centers in Indonesia and the Philippines. We attribute this success of breastfeeding to the enthusiastic way in which babies born at our birth centers bond wide-eyed and go directly to the breast to self-attach and feed. Delayed umbilical cord clamping and cutting makes it possible for babies to be bright and energetic. Babies subjected to immediate cord severance suffer from newborn anemia and all of their bonding and breastfeeding activities are impaired.

Severe anemia makes any and all newborn activities, such as gazing, crawling toward the breast, nuzzling, staying awake, latching and suckling, nearly impossible. I sing praises to the determined mothers who manage to bond and breastfeed their infants, in spite of immediate cord severance. Humans are super resilient, but that is no reason to abuse them at birth.

No other mammal, except humans, routinely interferes with bonding and breastfeeding by quickly severing the umbilical cords of their offspring.

My question:
If baby needs neonatal resuscitation is there a benefit to immediate cord cutting?

There is absolutely no need to immediately clamp and cut the baby's umbilical cord to facilitate neonatal resuscitation. In fact, the oxygen rich blood provided by the intact cord, helps the baby transition. There are now neonatal resuscitation units available and used by hospitals interested in optimal newborn care, which accommodate neonatal resuscitation right beside or above mother. Even without such a unit, the Bumi Sehat midwives, on frequent occasions, have successfully resuscitated stillborn babies right by the mother's side with umbilical cord still intact.[22]

My question:
Who suffers as a victim of this barbaric practice?

No matter if you are rich or poor; educated or not; brown, black, white, red, yellow or of mixed race; Muslim, Christian, Buddhist, Hindu, Pagan, Catholic, Jewish or Agnostic; very young or quite mature, if you go to a medical institution for childbirth, your baby will likely be robbed of up to ⅓ (33%) of his or her natural blood supply. Your child is in immediate danger at the time of birth of a cascading series of medical interventions and possible bonding issues as a direct result. Also, consider the long-term impact and complications to his/her physical, emotional and mental health, which can lead to overall detrimental impacts on society; and that means that all of us suffer from our folly.

My final question… for now:
What will it take for us to stand up for the integrity and sanctity of our children's birthright?

Just say "NO, I will not allow anyone to abuse my newborn by immediately clamping and cutting my Baby's umbilical cord!" It is your duty as a parent.

If you were born in a hospital or clinic, it happened to you. If you plan to give birth in nearly any medical institution on Earth, it will happen to your baby, unless YOU demand time for your baby to receive all of the blood he or she is meant to have.[23]

Immediate or early clamping and cutting of babies' umbilical cords is the most flagrantly widespread, medically sanctioned Human Rights issue on Earth! Together, we can make this a thing of the past. May our babies all be blessed by our patience, a patience needed to allow Mother Nature and Father Time to effect the perfect process for optimal gentle birth.

> *"CONCLUSION: Iron stores and Hb in infancy can be improved in neonates born to anemic mothers by delaying cord clamping at birth."*
>
> *~WHO/UNICEF Guidance on Management of the*
> *Third Stage of Labor and Timing of Cord Clamping:*
> *Are we throwing the baby out with the bath water?*
> *Complied by IYCFC Unit, Nutrition Section, UNICEF*
> *HQ, August 2003*

Is Homebirth Safe?

There are many variables, are you healthy? Is this pregnancy unfolding in a healthy, normal, natural way? Do you have skilled midwives, who are willing to provide you with the opportunity to birth at home? Is your home reasonably close to good back-up, should risks to you or your baby develop requiring transport to hospital? Discuss all of this with your midwives, If they agree with you, planning a homebirth is a reasonable idea.

Pregnancy and birth are not illnesses. Women should have the choice to give birth where they feel most safe, supported and comfortable. for some mothers-to-be, that is hospital, for others the choice could be a childbirth center, and for still others, HomeBirth is just right. Most of the time healthy mothers carrying a healthy baby, will not develop complications during labor. Midwives spend abundant time with mothers during prenatal care, screening for possible risks. Midwives also do not disrupt the natural process of labor and birth. When birth is not interfered with, the risks are lower, because our bodies know how to have babies.

In the Netherlands ⅓ of all mothers are birthing at home. In the United Kingdom the National Health Service (NHS) has proclaimed that; 40 to 45% of all mothers in the UK are healthy and low risk during pregnancy, and should deliver their babies at home. The UK provides skilled HomeBirth midwives, paid for by the NHS. These countries have better MotherBabyBirth outcomes than the United States of America, the country that spends the most on childbirth technology, tests and interventions. The USA currently ranks 60th out of 179 countries for maternal mortality. It is safer to birth in 59 countries.

If you are wishing for WatherBirth, freedom to choose how and with whom you birth, delayed clamping and cutting of your baby's umbilical cord, or lotus birth, it may be much easier to have these options respected, if you are at home, in the care of skilled midwives. Most hospitals have many procedures, rules and protocols, like a "One size fits all" kind of childbirth. If you want to eat sushi, you don't go to the hamburger café. If you want all your choices held in regard, if you believe in "MY Body, MY Birth, MY Baby… If you wish to be certain that you and Baby will be supported to have your First Embrace uninterrupted, stay healthy and stay home if you possibly can.

Safety of Midwife Care

According to a 2009 Cochrane meta-analysis of studies* (12,276 women) looking at midwife-led care versus care by an obstetrician or family physician, midwifery care was found to have as good or better outcomes in every parameter. Under midwife care women had less: need for anesthesia, episiotomies, instrumental birth (such as forceps or vacuum). Furthermore women had increased: feelings of control in labor, likelihood of spontaneous vaginal birth and successful breast-feeding. The researchers have found over and over that midwife-led care is associated with several benefits for mothers and babies, and had no identified adverse effects.*Hatem M, Sandall J, Devane D, Soltani H, Gates S.

Midwife-led versus other models of care for childbearing women. Cochrane Database of Systematic Reviews 2008, Issue 4.

WaterBirth...

Yes using warm water in labor and childbirth does reduce pain. When my 4th baby was born I had WaterBirth, and it was much less painful. This birth was so fast, I am very thankful that my midwives, Jan Francisco and Tina Garzero, coaxed me into the warm water tub they had prepared. Nice warm showers during labor, are a wonderful use of water therapy. If you have a midwife or doctor who is experienced in receiving babies in the water, and a birth tub is available, WaterBirth is a natural wonderful way of reducing pain and stress during labor and birth for both mom and baby.

Do not leave the baby under water. That is not to say, rush, once the baby's head is out, don't panic, let the baby's head turn naturally and the body will soon follow, with the next contraction. Your midwives (or your, yourself) will scoop the baby gently up to the surface and wait for you, the mother, to take the baby to your heart, and put him or her on your chest. Keep the baby's head on your chest, above the water line. Baby's body may still be submerged in the water, while his or her head and face are out of the water. Unless you leave baby submerged too long, baby will only take a first breath when his/her face is safely out of the water. This is called the "dive reflex."

Leave the umbilical cord intact and wait patiently for the placenta to be born. The baby may breastfeed right away, if the cord is long enough for him or her to reach mother's breasts. This helps the placenta come easily and prevents postpartum hemorrhage. There is no hurry. Cutting the umbilical cord in the water is foolish. Cutting the baby's umbilical cord is a sterile procedure, because to sever it in an unsterile way, is dangerous. There is no risk of infection if the umbilical cord is left intact.

Some midwives like to help the mother birth her placenta in a comfortable place, outside of the birth tub. If you deliver placenta in the tub, once the placenta is born you may gently rinse it clean while it is still in the tub and attached to baby, and float it in a bowl, keep baby warm. When you and baby are ready to get out, two people must hold baby and placenta, and move them to the bed. Keep baby warm and dry, and stay with baby. Two people must help you, mother to rinse off with clean water and slowly stand up, dry off and with help walk safely to the bed to lie down and breastfeed. Some mothers feel they are super strong, and can simply stand up, holding the baby and placenta in bowl and walk bravely to the bed. Well, it's better to be safe than to fall or slip down along the way. Yes ~ you are incredibly strong, and you just did the most amazing job on planet Earth, you birthed this baby... now, allow people to help you, please. Birth team: make very sure that there are towels on the floor, to prevent the mother from slipping when she emerges from the birth tub. Mother, if you feel very strong and clear, two or more people may help you to get out of tub, baby in arms, placenta in bowl, carried close by another person, and walk carefully to a nearby bed, or place prepared for MotherBaby to rest. Just don't march out of your birth tub all alone, it's unwise.

Water birth is a simple and natural method of reducing pain in labor. It is gentle and easy to do. Don't be disappointed if you planned water birth, then had to or wished to get out of the water to deliver the baby. This happens sometimes, the most important thing is that you and baby have the most gentle natural birth possible for you.

Right at the Time of Birth...

- Keep your baby with you, don't allow anyone to separate you from baby.

- Staying skin to skin with your baby is the very best.

- Sing a song of your Faith... a prayer, a mantra, a hymn to greet your baby.

- Keep your baby's umbilical cord intact. There is no need to cut it.

- Breastfeed as soon as possible. Exclusively breastfeed for at least 6 months.

- Your Baby's father, or you, may choose a special meaningful thing to say to the baby as a greeting, at birth, this sets the tone for a rich spiritual life for your child.

First Embrace

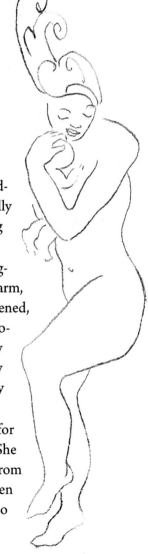

In the Philippines, my MotherLand, Mothers, Grand-mothers, Families, Midwives, nurses and doctors really are looking at a prioritizing something we call "Unang Yakap" ~ First Embrace.

Birth~ is that magical moment when baby emerges into the world, one moment she/he is in the warm, moist, dark womb, where sounds and light are softened, and the temperature is always perfect. Oxygen is provided and all circulatory functions are supported by the placenta. The process of birth itself is initiated by the baby. It can be long or short, but it is definitely something the baby is experiencing as a big change.

The next moment baby is OUT in the world... for the Baby birth can be a shocking traumatic event. She may feel cold for the first time. Imagine separation from umbilical cord, placenta, and the subsequent oxygen deprivation that can cause, if the cord is severed too soon.

Babies naturally grasp for mother, and mother should be right there, supported by her Birth team, to receive her baby.

Even if the baby needs resuscitation, there need not be a traumatic separation. Neonatal resuscitation can happen beside the mother, between her legs, or on a special NNR table that rolls right up to the birth bed, allowing Neonatal Resuscitation, close to mother, with intact umbilical cord, which is optimal for baby.

All too often the baby is born, within seconds the umbilical cord is clamped and cut and baby is taken away for drying, weighing, measuring, and warming. Guess what? Baby does not care what he weights. She/he only wants to be in the embrace of Mother, where Nature intended babies to be, Skin-to-Skin with the familiar warmth, welcoming voice and loving gaze of Mother. For an arriving baby, Mother is the Universe, the source of all love and nourishment.

Deborah Flowers says, "When the Baby is separated from mother, it's like s/he's landed on an alien planet."

Many people have described having the experience of being abducted by "Aliens." Again and again, these people paint the same scenario: A very large humanoid, five or six time her size, wearing a mask (sometimes also wearing glasses) carries her naked to a stainless steel, cold surface (scale) to weigh and measure her. Then a long glass tube, with a smooth metal tip (thermometer), is inserted into her anus, to detect and record body temperature. The huge people speak in loud voices, a language the victim cannot understand. The lights are too bright, hurting the eyes. Sounds are too loud and harm the ears. The room is too open and huge, causing the being to feel vulnerable, afraid. This scenario, described almost word for word, by most people who feel they were abducted by aliens, is exactly what happens to a newborn baby, when s/he is born in a hospital. For far too many newborn babies, birth is a traumatic experience of separation, feelings of abandonment, having been abducted by aliens, transported to an alien planet.

Optimal First embrace:

Baby emerges gently, no pulling on her body. When birth is unfolding in health, there is no hurry, no worry. Next... Mother reaches for her Baby, no one interferes. No one shouts: "It's a Boy." or "It's a Girl!"

The mother may need a moment or moments, before embracing her baby. As Baby transitions from Womb life, to Earth life, Mother is transitioning from being pregnant to having a newborn in her arms. Once the new mother, reaches for her baby, and enfold her/him in the first warm, protective, bonding embrace... well, it's a miracle, the most profound of love pours forth, from all concerned.

Pregnant Pause: Many mothers are shy, they will look at Baby in awe, look at their partner, look back at Baby, Touch Baby tenderly... and eventually, take baby in her own hands, and hug her to her heart. What an empowering moment!

Skin-to-skin the Mother and Baby, and family may bond, and initiate breastfeeding. This is a sacred bubble, and except in the case of a dire emergency, this bubble of First Embrace must be respected.

The research proves that the first embrace at the time of birth, with skin to skin contact is so important for:

- The success of Breastfeeding (and duration of breastfeeding)
- Kangaroo Care for better weight gain and survival of premature babies.
- Healthy Babies who are born by Cesarean may enjoy that first embrace, and skin-to-skin bonding with mother, quite soon after birth by cesarean.
- Many health care practitioners are unaware of the positive effects of skin-to-skin MotherBaby bonding, and their care reflects this lack of knowledge. Healthcare practitioners involved in caesarean procedures, need better education concerning what Babies need.

Where you give birth and with whom, will certainly determine weather or not you and baby get to have that First Embrace.

Too many mothers say: "I was in the Hospital, and one thing led to another. I ended up with a cesarean. My Baby and I never did get to have that First Embrace."

Even the case of prematurity ~ Babies should not be routinely separated from mother. They should not routinely have their umbilical cords clamped and cut.

The mother's body regulates the baby's temperature better than an incubator can. Premie babies belong skin-to-skin.

The mother's colostrum and milk, nourish and hydrate, even the tiny fragile baby, better than IV fluids can.

Unang Yakap ~ First Embrace, Skin-to-skin contact for MotherBaby is optimal, evidenced based care. Ask for it, expect it as the triumph of your birthing. It is your human right, and your baby's human right.

The Father's or Other Mother's Job at Birth....

note: If you are in a same-sex relationship, this job is equally important for Baby's other mother. If you don't have a "father" for your child, choose someone who loves MotherBaby, to do this. Mother can also do this, but she is quite occupied at the moment of birth, and may not remember.

I ask the father or mother's partner to choose something significant and sacred to say or sing to the baby, as the first thing baby shall hear upon arrival Earth-side.

This is because I believe (and many Faiths teach this) that when we die, even if we live to be over 100 years, all of our life experiences will be remembered by our soul. Each detail, especially the most significant and tender of our life events, will be reviewed by each of us. Hearing is such an acute sense at birth, and at death. Even deaf people who have died and come back claim to have "heard" things they needed to know. It is believed in many cultures that the first thing a newborn baby hears at birth, will be the last thing he or she remembers of this world, when passing over. This is why I ask for the first thing each baby hears at birth to be something intentionally chosen, to open and close the circle of life.

I am not sure what my husband said to our youngest son, when he slipped from my body, into his father's hands, it is their secret. I do think I heard something about, Love, and Music… this boy is a gifted musician, very loving, diligent and spiritual in his day to day approach to life. It is reassuring as he navigates the storms of his young life, that he had the most gentle, loving, intentional start at birth.

Should our Baby's Mother or Father, or other Parent Cut the Cord?

If you have read most of this book already, you know that I don't at all agree with immediate or too soon-after-birth umbilical cord clamping and cutting. It has become a "thing" to immediately clamp the cord in the moments following the baby's emergence from the mother's yoni, and hand the scissors to the baby's father (or mother's partner) asking, "Do you want to cut the cord?"

There is something very wrong with this practice. First of all, it all happens too fast, before baby gets her or his full blood supply and stem cell transfusion from the placenta. Secondly, when the baby's father (or other parent) cuts the cord, he/she becomes the person who severs the life-link, destroying the sacred trinity of Baby, cord and Placenta. I feel this is NOT a nice introduction into Parenthood.

Intuitively and instinctually the new mother knows it is her life-partner's job, to protect this new baby. Even if she has not thought about the timing of umbilical cord severance, when she sees it happen, she feels it is not right. The new mother may never consciously think it or say it, but when the baby's father or other parent cuts the cord, something is severed, and her trust of this person is damaged.

New Papa or Mama, it is not your job to cut or sever the cord. Your job is to protect this tiny baby given into your care. Your partner has worked so diligently to bring the baby to Earth, do not shatter her trust for you, buy making a ritual of cord severance, please, even if the doctor offers you the dubious honor.

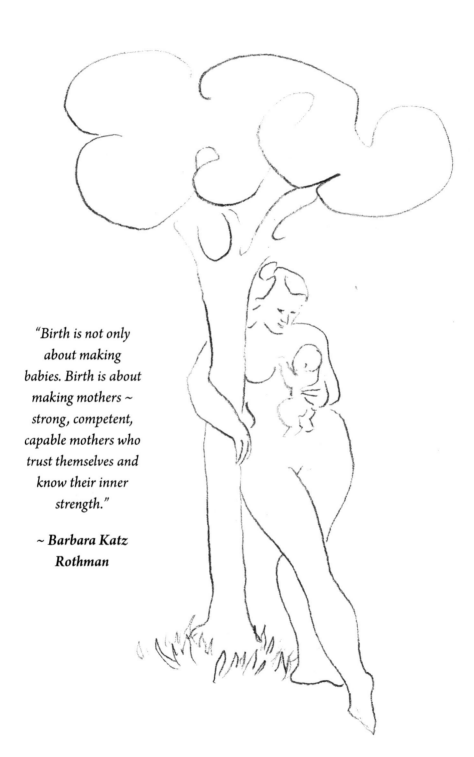

"Birth is not only about making babies. Birth is about making mothers ~ strong, competent, capable mothers who trust themselves and know their inner strength."

~ *Barbara Katz Rothman*

The First 24 Hours Postpartum

I recommend that for the first 24 hours following childbirth, the new MotherBaby should never be left entirely alone. Also, MotherBaby should never be separated, but kept skin-to-skin. For the first few hours a healthcare provider, midwife and or nurse, should be nearby. This is especially important if the mother has lost a significant amount of blood. After the first few hours, family members and close female friends/sisStars, should be nearby. Even if mother and baby look and feel good, staying close is a perfect way to insure nothing goes left, unnoticed. When mother goes to the toilet, to prevent falling and fainting, someone should accompany her. It can happen in a moment, the new mother's body is in a time of immense adjustment from pregnancy to postpartum. Her hormones went from high above normal levels to 50% below normal. Her blood volume is much reduced, her blood pressure may be lower. Plus, she is on cloud 9 (as my mOM would say)... she's in a bubble of baby bliss and must be looked after and protected. It is the family's honor and privilege to stay continuously beside the new MotherBaby, their glow is something truly divine.

Baby's Placenta... What now?

The placenta is the original tree of life. She is a mythical Gorgon that keeps mother and baby alive during the long weeks of gestation. Placenta is Ganesh the protector of families, the eight-armed Durga riding a tiger helping the mother bring her baby Earth-side. Placenta is the forgotten chakra, the physical body of baby's guardian Angel, made from scratch, by love. One thing I know in my heart, the placenta is not medical waste.

Make sure that if you birth in the hospital that they have a provision for you to take home your baby's placenta for a respectful burial. The Balinese people believe that the placenta is the body of your child's guardian angel. In Indonesia no hospital would dare to keep the placenta from the family, of they tried the baby's people would burn the hospital down!

Once you get the placenta home, or if you are already at home, you may wish to encapsulate it. There are many reasons to do this, and you can read up on it and arrange for placenta encapsulation before your baby's birth

Handing the placenta is the father, or other Mother's job. The birth mother's job is to rest and breastfeed. The most simple way to bless placenta on to the afterlife is to bury it, either in a special place in your garden, or in a big pot with a tree planted with it. this is a good option if you may be moving. You can simply bring the pot with you to your new home. Once you settle into a permanent home, plant the tree. Your child will love growing up with his or her tree, a place to play, some trees give fruit, others colorful leaves, all give shade.

... for much more information about all aspects of placenta please read my book: "Placenta the Forgotten Chakra."

Circumcision...

I nearly skipped this subject, because there is so much charge around it. Circumcision is NOT just a harmless snip. Circumcision both male and female are done for cosmetic reasons, to alter the way the child's genitals will look. Most surgeries are chosen, or not chosen, based on an assessment of benefits verses risks. There are NO benefits of circumcision, and many profound risks. The researcher Dan Bollinger concluded that about 117 neonatal deaths of baby boys occur in the United States of America, per year, due directly or indirectly to circumcision.[24] Imagine the grief! My own nephew was circumcised in the hospital, before release, my sister never gave consent. She was handed the baby by a nervous staff nurse and hurried out the door. She noticed while driving home that her baby, safely strapped into the infant car seat, in the back, looked pale and unwell. She went directly to her family pediatrician. They found my nephew's diaper was soaked through with blood. The doctor who did the circumcision had removed part of the head of baby Brian's penis, along wit his foreskin. During Brian's first year of life, he suffered five more major corrective surgeries. His first sentence was, "Mommy, my penis hurt."

If you are considering circumcision because your baby's father is circumcised, and you want them to look the same down stairs, they will not. Grown men generally have a lot of pubic hair, while small boys have none. My sons, I have four, never noticed that dad was circumcised and they all had foreskins. They noticed that dad was hairy and they were not. My sons are now grown and they have never suffered from problems caused by being uncircumcised. My grandsons are also intact. All the females and males in my family are uncircumcised.

There are many myths concerning the benefits of circumcision. It has never been proven to be effective in either reducing or treating cervical cancer, penile cancer, urinary tract infections, or sexually transmitted diseases including HIV/AIDS.[25] Not one medical association in America, or anywhere else in the world, recommends infant circumcision; and some recommend against circumcision.[26] At no time in its 75 years has the American Academy of Pediatrics ever recommended infant circumcision.

Circumcision hurts,[27] it severs over 1,000 nerves, in the most sensitive area of the body. There are so many reasons to NOT circumcise your baby. Babies cannot speak for themselves. We must protect them from needless harm, regardless of your culture or personal taste. Circumcision is a decision you cannot undo. For more information and facts, look for the Circumcision DECISION-MAKER, on line: circumcisiondecisionmaker.com

Sleeping with Baby...

Mammals sleep with their babies. I could not imagine putting my babies in a crib. I was given a crib, which I only tired one time, when baby was four months old. Moments after laying her asleep in the crib, she woke and cried, and to see her behind bars, just shattered my heart. So, we continued to sleep together, no matter what people said. You will need to make your own decision about sleeping with baby. Follow your heart, your own inner knowing. Read all there is to find out there.

There are bedside co-sleeper attachments. They are much more MotherBaby friendly than a crib.

Some good safety tips for sleeping with Baby...

- Check all around your bed to make sure there are no crevices where baby could become dangerously stuck. Sleeping with Baby is best when the bed is big and wide, like king or queen sized. If your bed is very high, lower it. I put my mattress on the floor for the first two to three years of each of my babies' lives, to prevent falling out of bed, once they began to roll over.

- It is safer for baby to sleep on his or her back. When breastfeeding in bed, roll to your side, get really comfortable, bring baby close, on her/his side, so you are belly-to-belly, if baby has to twist her/his neck to get to your nipple, you are not in a good position yet. Usually, after baby feeds, she/he will roll back over on her/his back. You can encourage this safer sleeping position.

- Studies show that sleeping with baby beside mother, but not between mother and her partner, is safer.

- Keep soft cushions and big billowy quilts away form your sleeping baby.

Do not sleep with your baby under these circumstances:

- Do not sleep with baby if you are under the influence of any substance or drug (such as alcohol or tranquilizing medications) these substances will diminish your sensitivity to baby's presence. If you are drunk or drugged, you are less-able to be aroused from sleep, should baby need you or be in danger. Under the influence of drugs or alcohol, parents are more likely to roll over onto or step on baby.

- Do not sleep with baby if you are extremely overweight. Obesity itself may cause mother to suffer from sleep apnea. This can lead to an exhausted mother, who is more likely to roll onto baby, so there is risk of smothering. A Co-sleeper works very well for larger moms.

- Do not sleep with baby if you are suffering from sleep deprivation. Exhaustion lessens awareness of your baby and reduces your ability to wake up and be available for your baby. It is best to try to nap in the daytime, when baby is sleeping, to avoid exhaustion.

- Do not breastfeed baby, and fall asleep, laying down on a squishy, cushiony or "sinky" surface, such as a waterbed or couch. An exhausted mother could fall asleep breastfeeding and roll over on the baby. There is danger if baby becomes wedged between back of couch and a sleeping bigger person. Waterbeds pose a danger of suffocation for babies.

- Don't allow your child's baby-sitter to sleep with baby. A baby-sitter's awareness and arousability are unlikely to be as acute as a mother's. Also, don't lay baby down ob a bed, with another sleeping person, who is unaware of baby's presence.

- Don't allow older siblings to sleep with a baby under nine months. Sleeping children do not have the same awareness of tiny babies as do parents, Keep in mind, a crowded bed space is not a good arrangement for co-sleeping safely. Babies are safest sleeping beside their mothers.

- Don't over-bundle baby. Your warm body is an added heat source. Make sure your baby's chest is covered with an appropriate baby t-shirt, so that if she or he sweats at night, s/he won't get a chill.

- Never cover baby's head.

- Don't wear lingerie with string ties longer than 6 to 8 inches. Avoid dangling jewelry and loose necklaces, they could entangle baby.

- Avoid all pungent, unnatural hair sprays, deodorants, and perfumes, laundry detergent, powders, etc. They camouflage and interfere with the natural maternal smells that soothe baby. Foreign odors may irritate and clog baby's tiny nasal passages. Second hands smoke, is very bad for Baby.

- Use common sense when co-sleeping safely. Remember, Anything that could cause you to sleep more soundly than usual or that alters your consciousness can affect your baby's safety. Nearly all the suspected (but seldom proven) cases of fatal "overlying" found in the medical literature could have been avoided. Observe common sense sleeping practices.

BabyMoon

Most ancient and indigenous cultures allow for a sacred laying-in time of 42 days postpartum for mothers to rest, recover from childbirth, be served and revered, while they bond and breastfeed new Baby. I call this your "BabyMoon."

Dangers of the WIND

Oriental traditions of medicine teach that the new MotherBaby must be protected from "masuk angin" the wind entering their bodies can make them unwell and or cranky/ill tempered. To prevent this, new mothers eat warm easy to digest foods, they stay at home, or in the quiet of a warm sunny garden. MotherBaby dress in warm, not too hot clothing, and stay skin-to-skin by opening the front of their garments, laying baby upon mother's breasts. MotherBaby must be protected from loud sounds, pollution and arguing. Only people with good loving intentions may visit. Electronic devices and gadgets should be used sparingly. Do not keep a hand phone beside your sleeping baby. Anything that stirs a violent wind should be avoided. If the baby goes out of the home, his or her fontanel (soft spot) should be covered, a small hat will do, to protect from the wind or bad vibrations entering. Protecting new MotherBaby from the wind entering their very vulnerable bodies is all part of the family's responsibility during the BabyMoon.

The first few days are the most sacred and should be undisturbed. Remember childbirth has washed the mother's body and soul clean. The baby is brand-new from heaven (Yes ~ I believe Heaven is the inside of a woman's womb!)

I remember when my daughter was in her first day postpartum, after her amazing gentle home lotus birth, people came and expected her musician husband to come away with them on a film shoot. Arrangements had been tentative, and the producer knew the couple was expecting a baby any minute. My son-in-love was upset, he did not want to leave the bubble of his Baby's Birth, he did not wish to leave his wife, even for a few hours, but the producer was aggressive.

I intervened, "Would you expect this man to leave his Honey Moon bed, to do a shoot for you today?" I asked.

"Of course not!" was her reply, "We would respect his Honey Moon." I explained that the BabyMoon was much more important and should be at least equally respected. She did not see it my way. I feel sad and sorry for this woman, who puts business above new babies. She is painfully closed hearted.

During the 42 sacred BabyMoon days postpartum mothers should stay home. They should be fed delicious foods, and given nutritious drinks, to hydrate them for ample milk supply. They should have postpartum massages, with warm oil. There is more wonderful advice in the Ayurvedic pages of this book.

Mother, while you are looking after and nurturing your Baby, something magical happens. The family comes together, and functions in a bubble of increasing love. Mothers, know that by giving yourself this time, to be supported, and nourished, you nurture your creative, deepest, most authentic self. ALL kinds of miracles begin to occur. Your Creative Intelligence will be enlivened by the hormones of breastfeeding. The days and nights of exclusively caring for Baby will evolve into an Awakening of your creativity. This process happens best, when a proper 42 day BabyMoon is honored by the family. Unfortunately, most societies do not yet honor a proper BabyMoon. It is our time in herstory, to reinvent humanity, to be MORE HUMAN. BabyMoon, Conscious Conception, Gentle Childbirth, Exclusive Breastfeeding... are all part of this evolution.

If you are forced by circumstance, to return to the work-a-day world, before you have had a proper BabyMoon, please get a good quality breast pump, and take the time and space, to keep your milk flow going. When you arrive home, wash off the outside world, with a quick shower. Next, hug your baby skin-to-skin, to reestablish your special bond. You may find this is a time of deep breathing, and some tears, and long loving breastfeeding.

"Babies are bits of star-dust blown from the hand of God. Lucky the woman who knows the pangs of birth for she has held a star." ~ *Larry Barretto*

Breastfeeding

the Art of Getting Started...

First of all remember that it takes all human mothers two to three days (maybe more if she is nutritionally depleted or has other stress) for her milk to come in (arrive). This means it is extremely important that you feed your baby ONLY at the breast. Baby's sucking stimulates the breasts to manufacture and deliver milk more quickly and efficiently. Also, your baby needs the first milk, called colostrum, which is yellow, and comes out in small but sufficient amounts before the true milk flows. It is dangerous and unwise to wait to put the baby to the breast, just because the milk is not yet flowing. Please don't get talked into giving the baby bottles of infant formula, just because your milk is not yet flowing. Most babies do lose a bit of weight, in the first few days of life, this is normal. Prevailing with exclusive breastfeeding, whenever your baby wants to nurse, is the best way to help your baby stay well hydrated, and gain some weight. Newborn humans have 5% brown adipose tissue, also know as "Brown Fat" to help them stay warm and survive the first few transition days of life on Earth. Your breast milk, delivered at the perfect temperature, and formulated by your body, exactly as your baby needs it, is all your baby needs for the first 6 months of life.

Remember that the belly of a newborn baby is very tiny, and cannot hold more than a few drops of colostrum at birth. If you feed her or him a bottle of cow's milk formula, the baby's belly will hurt. The baby will suck the easy-flowing milk from the bottle, because babies are born thirsty and they are born with the urge to suck a lot. This is so they can help their mother's milk come in, as nature intended it, in increments, not to fast, but just right for baby's belly capacity. Also, ask yourself, do I want my newborn baby to be ingesting the stem cells of cows? Mother's milk, be it human, panda or cow, is full of stem cells. Human milk is medicine as well as nourishment, for humans. Some infant formula contains soymilk, which has been found to be made from genetically engineered soybeans.

Breastfeeding is BEST-feeding... Things that help milk flow:

- Relaxing, resting
- Getting the baby well on the breast as soon as possible after birth
- Breastfeeding the baby often, for long periods of time on both sides
- Eat plenty of green leafy vegetables and red rice porridge.
- EAT well.
- Drink plenty of pure water and nutritious fluids, like orange juice.
- Do NOT give baby a bottle of water, nor infant formula, it will hurt him/her.
- Don't believe the good things advertized about infant formula, remember in some parts of the world hospitals, doctors and even midwives are in business to promote infant formula. If they can get your baby hooked on their product, you essentially work for them, spending heaps of money, every month to buy their milk, which is far inferior to your own breastmilk.
- Mother's milk is free, and immeasurably more healthy.
- Make sure your baby opens his mouth wide to take in the nipple and much of the areola breast tissue.
- If you come to bumps in the road on the way to easy breastfeeding, please don't get discouraged. La Leche League International (LLL) is an organization that has helpful people, willing to answer the phone and give you correct advice, some can come and help you. There are LLL meetings in most majoy cities in the USA, check your phone book for their listing. You can reach out to experienced mothers for help. Your midwives and doulas are willing to help you, they care about breastfeeding, please don't be shy to ask.

A good way to initiate breastfeeding is will baby right up on top of you, in any position that you find comfortable, considering that you have just given birth. Most babies will begin to bob their heads and inch their way to your breasts. Some mothers wish to wait and let baby find the way, which can take more than an hour. I could not contain my joy, and I scooped each of my babies closer to my breasts, so they could immediately latch on.

When getting started, another way to breastfeed lying down is to lie on your side, bring the baby close, also lying on his or her side. Make sure the baby is not on his back, which will cause him to strain and twist his neck, just to get to the nipple. A good guideline is to look at baby's head, neck and spine, they should be in a nice straight line while feeding, not twisted to one side or the other.

When sitting-up breastfeeding, remember to keep the baby turned towards you. Your family may help by bringing a pillow for your lap, to put the baby up onto, so the mother does not need to bend and strain her upper back, while feeding. Again, check to see that baby's neck is nice and straight, not twisted, straining to get well-on your breast. The baby's mouth should open nice and wide, and he or she should latch on to more than just your nipple, but a good amount of the surrounding areola. If baby is sucking just your nipple, you will become sore, and baby will not be satisfied. Gently reposition baby and coax him or her to open wide, before latching on. Gentle strokes of your finger on baby's cheek usually will do the trick of getting the mouth wide open.

Fathers/partners may also help bring the new mother nice drinks of water, or juice or something nutritious that she enjoys, while she is breastfeeding. I loved young coconut water. Remember that you will need extra nutrition and hydration while you are making milk.

My body knows how to make perfect milk, delivered at the perfect temperature, in the prefect amount that my baby needs.

Mother's Milk, Supply and Demand....

Remember that it is the baby's sucking at the breasts that stimulate the production of milk. Every time a baby is bottle fed, his mother will produce less milk for the next day. This is a vicious cycle.

Modern humans are inundated with ads, which promote bottle feeding. Your extended family has also seen these ads, and they may push you to bottle feed. It is up to you to stay calm and firm in your resolve to exclusively breastfeed your baby.

The breastfeeding family is under less financial strain, therefore breastfeeding mothers are more liberated than the bottle feeding moms. Breastfed babies are sick far less than bottle fed babies, so breastfed babies experience fewer trips to the doctors, and less exposure to pharmaceutical medicine (with all its side effects). Who says breastfeeding is old fashioned? Clearly it is more natural, and clearly it is the most intelligent choice. Don't let society convince you to bottle feed. Remember it is you who must bear the costs of bottle feeding. It is you who will need to walk to the kitchen and prepare bottles in the middle of the night, if you bottle feed. Breastfeeding moms need only roll over in bed and give their breast to the baby to suckle.

It is your baby, your entire family and society who will reap the benefits of breastfeeding. Therefore we must trust exclusive breastfeeding as the most healthy, natural, hygienic, and economic way to feed babies for the first six months of life.

Painful Engorged Breasts

Usually when a new mother calls me to say; "My breasts are painfully hard and I don't know what to do." she has become over tired, a bit dehydrated, and has most likely gone out of her home, and done too much, the day before.

The Best Remedy for Painfully Engorged Breasts:

- Grate fresh ginger root, put it in a bowl.
- Pour hot water on the ginger.
- Soak a clean white cloth in this ginger concoction, to make a hot compress.
- Compress each breast several times, as hot as possible, without burning yourself.
- Stay in bed and sleep when your baby sleeps. Exhausted mothers are more likely to get engorged breasts.

Continue to breastfeed your baby as often as possible, beginning on the most engorged breast. This keeps your milk flowing and avoids mastitis, which means infected breasts. Don't believe anyone who tells you to stop breastfeeding. You need to feed your baby when you are engorged, and your baby needs your milk. It is perfectly fine to keep breastfeeding, in fact it is dangerous to stop.

"Nursing does not diminish the beauty of a woman's breasts; it enhances their charm by making them look lived in and happy." ~ Robert A. Heinlein

Cesarean Birth

Sometimes the best of plans, do not work out. Having a cesarean does not mean you did not give birth. Your unique birth experiences should not be discounted because it did not happen all naturally. Too often stress caused by disappointment compromises the success of breastfeeding. Don't let sadness and disappointment rob you of the joy of mothering. It's a challenging enough job, without guilt added to the stew.

I have attended cesarean births that were necessary and so beautiful. A skilled surgical team is most important. Our back-up surgeons in Bali are very respectful and understanding, they even sing Gayatri Mantra or the Muslim Azahn or Christian hymns with us, when the baby is actually being born. We believe the mother and the baby benefit from this gentle respect.

Your focus now is on being a mother. Take joy in your baby. Have a lot of good cries, preferably in the arms of a dear and understanding friend or sisStar. Don't guilt-trip yourself. If you feel angry or disappointed, please don't let negative emotions drive a wedge between you and your bliss. Cesarean birth, is birth a different kind of miracle.

VBAC, Vaginal Birth After Cesarean:

If you have already had a cesarean birth, there is no reason to plan for another. Vaginal birth after cesarean (VBAC) is generally safer than a repeat cesarean.

VBAC may be perceived as a risk, remember, having a baby at all carries some risk. This is why Mothers are so brave. Any kind of birth requires courage and support. The main risk does not lie in uterine rupture, which is extremely rare, of most concern is the psychological and spiritual stress of not going along with the powerful medical system.

Many brave families have blazed the trail. You should be able to find a midwife or doctor who is supportive. It may be challenging, but keep on trying until you feel you've found the one you trust.

Sofi's Vaginal Birth after Cesarean...

Sofi planned a natural birth, but her baby was in a transverse position when she went into labor. With the baby lying sideways, it was necessary for Sofi to have a cesarean birth. She was fortunate, she saw her baby immediately after the surgery, and the midwife helped her to initiate breastfeeding.

Three years later, when she was again pregnant Sofi at first had trouble finding someone to agree to support her in having a normal birth. Finally a friend told her about a midwife, who worked with a good back-up Obgyn doctor. After checking Sofi regularly, finding her to be in good health, the doctor and midwife agreed that she should plan for natural childbirth. Her midwife pointed out the fact that by breasfeeding her first child, Sofi had plenty of Oxytocin hormone receptors to help her future births go well. Oxytocin is monogamous with its own receptors, so the more love you give and share, the more capacity you have to LOVE!

Sofi came into the birth center 3 cm. dilated. She labored walking, hands and knees, and if tired she would rest on her left side. Her husband was a wonderful labor support. He made sure she drank and ate well to stay hydrated and to keep up her strength. Sofi's three-year-old son played nicely with the toys at the birth center, and awaited the birth of his sibling. Sometimes he crawled into his laboring mothers arms, and shared his own special support. A few hours later, to Sofi's surprise she was feeling like pushing. The midwife checked her and she was fully dilated. Sofi's husband held her from behind and she began to push. As the baby's head began to peek into view, Sofi's husband sang the Azahn, the song of his culture. He had tears in his eyes, to witness the miracle of birth.

The baby girl was 3.5 kilograms, 600 grams bigger than Sofi's first baby. She was born totally naturally. Sofi did have a small vaginal tear, which the midwife numbed with Lidocaine and sutured while the new baby breastfed. Afterward Sofi expressed how healing it was to finally have her dream come true, a natural, normal, gentle birth.

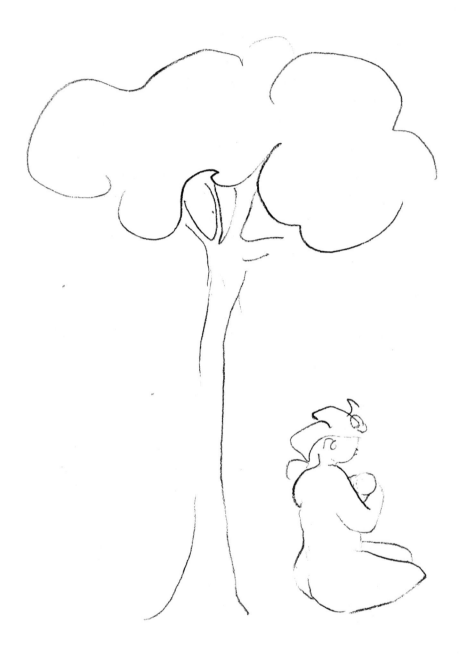

Postpartum

"You are pregnant for nine months, you're postpartum for the rest of your life." ~ Robin Lim

After our babies are born we mothers are as if in a special bubble, outside of time and space. It is a time for healing and rebuilding the deep strength of the mother's body. It is a time for bonding and establishing breastfeeding. It is MotherBabyMoon time.

In Sweden motherhood is so respected that postpartum women are given two years of maternity leave, with full pay. Naturally Sweden is among the countries with the lowest maternal and infant mortally rates in the world.

Use this sacred postpartum time to rest and rejoice. You should not plan any outside activities. Just stay home with the baby, let family and friends help you with day-to-day household duties, like cooking and laundry. While resting you may move around the house and garden, get fresh air to promote healing. After the first six weeks, add some light exercise, like yoga, swimming or dancing. There are some postpartum exercises suggested in this book. Traditional massages and belly wraps can be a wonderful way to enhance the benefits of your postpartum time. If you can get a postpartum doula to help you, I highly recommend one. Doulas are just amazing.

In Bali postpartum women are advised not to wash their hair or enter their kitchen, until the baby's umbilical cord stump has dried and fallen off. Not shampooing keeps wind and chills from getting into the postpartum mother, and staying out of the kitchen makes her sure to rest.

There is postpartum Jamu available in Indonesia. The most important ingredient is Turmeric. This is new-mother-medicine, to help you spring back and keep your sparkle after childbirth.

Turmeric Jamu

Ask your closest woman family member or friend to make this up for you while you are in labor, or anytime after childbirth. You can drink it during the first few days and weeks postpartum. The turmeric is anti bacterial, preventing infections, it is full of vitamins and minerals and it is a blood purifier and blood builder. The vitamin C in the limes promotes fast healing. Honey and tamarind are traditional medicines to balance your body. Honey is a tonic. Tamarind warms the body system and acts as a natural laxative. This will help your milk come in stronger and of better quality.

- ¼ kilo fresh turmeric – wash peel grate, kneed in pure water to extract juice, strain.

- Juice of 4 to 6 limes

- 1/8 kilo tamarind paste – seeds and shells strained out, kneed in pure water. Or look for Tamarind powder in health food stores. If you cannot find it, no worries.

- ½ cup natural real honey

- ½ tsp. sea salt

Combine all of the above adding water to make about 1 liter of Jamu. Keep refrigerated, shake well before each serving. Drink as desired. This Jamu will help make your body smell very good too.

Note: Traditionally in Indonesia women eat papaya during the days postpartum, to nourish their bodies, promote beauty and regular evacuation of the bowels.

Postpartum Exercises

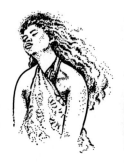

The Neck

Gently roll your neck in a complete circle, first one direction and then the other. Feel it lengthen, getting stronger. Feel any tension you may be holding float away.

Releasing the Neck and Upper Back

Supported by your elbows, which are aligned directly under the shoulders, stretch out facing skyward. Place your hands on either side of your bottom and let your head fall back gently. Feel the stretch in the front of your body and try to feel the shape of your upper back.

Lying flat, clasp your fingers together and cup your hands behind your head. Gently draw your elbows together; raise your shoulders slightly off the floor and roll your head forward, keeping your lower back pressed to the ground.

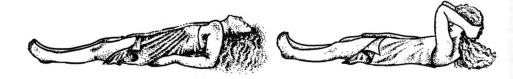

The Arms

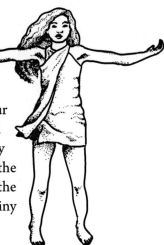

Stand with your feet shoulder width apart. Hold your arms out to the sides at shoulder level. Your palms are turned up as if you are receiving the sky. Let your neck be long. Your shoulders are down (not up around your ears) and arms are soft, rather than held stiffly. Inscribe tiny circles with the tips of your fingers. Slowly, increase the size of the circles until they are gigantic. Reverse the direction of the circles and gradually make them tiny again.

The Torso

Sit comfortably on the floor with your knees bent and the soles of your feet together. Draw your heels up close to you. Let your chin curl and your shoulders round as you allow the top of your head to drop forward.

Stretch your right arm over your head and reach to the left. Stretch your left arm over your head and reach to the right. You can feel the stretch in your torso with your opposite hand. Be sure to keep both your buttocks planted firmly on the ground, so you attain an optimum stretch.

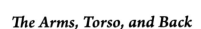

The Arms, Torso, and Back

Stand with your feet shoulder width apart; your knees are soft. Stretch your right arm over your left side, supporting yourself by placing your left hand at or slightly above knee level on the outside of your left leg. Feel the stretch from the arch of your right foot, through the leg, waist, arm, and all the way to the finger-tips. Hold the stretch as long as you like, the longer the better.

Now bend your knees and allow your right arm to drop and cross in front of you in a giant half circle. Exhale vigorously, making a swishing sound with your breath. Repeat on your left side.

Tai Chi Warm-Up

While standing with your feet shoulder width apart, raise both arms in front of you to shoulder level. Let them be soft. Bend your knees slightly, keeping them soft. Twist your entire upper body as if you are attempting to look behind you. Do not hold this position; allow yourself to unwind in the opposite direction. Your arms will follow behind; you want them so loose they feel as if they're boneless. Twist in one direction and then immediately go the other direction, as if it were one continuous movement. Breathe deeply.

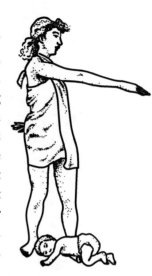

The Buttocks

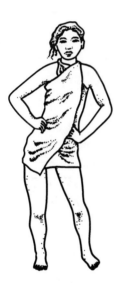

Stand with your knees soft and your feet shoulder width apart. Imagine you are standing inside an almost empty jar of peanut butter. You are going to scrape the insides of that jar with your *okole* (Hawaiian word for buttocks) so you can get the last of that delicious peanut butter. Circle your bot-tom and hips in one direction, then the other. You can put your hands on your hips.

Try doing kegel exercises while you do this toner. Now try inscribing a figure eight inside the jar with your hips.

From Head to Toe

Stand with feet shoulder width apart.

Relax everything.

Now shake every part of your body.

Allow a "haaaaaa" sound
to come from deep within.

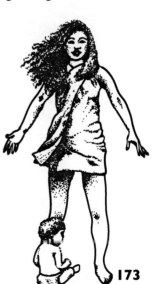

Now for the Legs

Stretch out on your side, propped up on your elbow. Cross your upper leg over the leg that is closest to the floor. Grip the ankle of the crossed leg. Flex the foot of your outstretched leg. Make sure your inner thigh is facing the ceiling. Now lift, lift, lift, lift the foot of your outstretched leg. The lift need not be large to feel the work in your inner thigh. Try not to let the foot touch the floor between lifts.

Roll over and do the same number of repetitions on the other side. Do kegel exercises while you are lifting, lifting, lifting.

The Toes and Feet

While in a squatting position with your palms on the floor in front of you, roll onto the balls of your feet. Dig your toes into the rug. Settle your weight back onto your heels and move your hands behind you, letting them take your weight. Curl your toes, stretching the tops of your feet. Wiggle your toes.

Swimming

Water is nature's revitalizer. Take every opportunity you can to swim. Feel the water wash away worry and fatigue. Feel the stretch and strength of each stroke. Feel the buoyancy of your body as it is cradled by the water. Introduce your baby to the water when he's in the mood. He'll love it if you do not force him and he feels safe.

Halloween Cat

This is another good exercise for relieving "mother's backache"; you also strengthen your back while you relax these muscles.

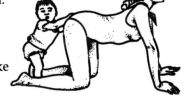

- Get onto hands and knees. Baby does whatever he or she wants to do.

- Exhale as you arch your spine toward the sky by tucking under head and bottom.

- Hold.

- Inhale as you release the position, letting your back relax. Don't allow back to sag like an old horse and do not force or press it toward the floor.

- Repeat as often as you like when your lower back needs a good stretch. Let your movement be fluid.

- During pregnancy, be extra conscious of concentrating on the upward movement. The extra weight of pregnancy already curves the back, which shortens the muscles in the area of the lower spine, so release from the arch gently. Even when not pregnant, the emphasis is on the upward stretch.

Pony Ride

This ride is great fun for baby and will tighten and strengthen your buttocks and thighs. Wait until your baby is two months old to do this one; before that age, many children may not enjoy this movement.

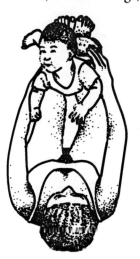

- To begin, lie on your back with your upper legs at a right angle to your torso. Your baby, lying tummy down, is balanced on your shins.

- When baby is comfortable, gently give him a ride up and down by raising and lowering your feet about six inches each way. Be sure to hold him carefully (Singing a silly song while doing the Pony Ride is very important.)

- Be very careful not to put strain on your knees.

Seat Walks

This movement will slim your thighs and tone your buttocks.

- Sit on the floor with your legs extended in front of you.

- Rock back and forth on your buttocks, reaching with your right hand while "walking" your right foot forward. Then, reach with your left hand while "walking" your left foot forward. In this way, seat-walk across the room.

- Moving backward, seat-walk yourself back to starting place.

- Accentuating the movement of your arms back and forth will make this exercise more beneficial, engaging and strengthening your torso and tummy while tightening your upper arms.

- Repeat as desired.

Out and Cross

While you are on the floor stretching your legs, roll onto your back. Gently rub your calves and thighs to warm your muscles. You will tone your inner thighs and buttocks with this exercise.

- While lying on the floor, let gravity gently pull your legs apart.

- Close and open your legs like a pair of scissors. (Do this with your feet flexed, then do it with your toes pointed.)

- Repeat daily and increase the number of repetitions as your strength improves.

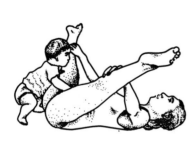

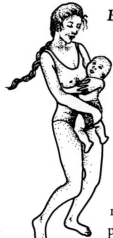

Baby Boogie

If you are in a playful mood, put on your favorite upbeat music. If you are feeling quiet, put on something classical. Be sensitive to your baby's mood also when you choose the music. There is no starting position, nor do I suggest any specific action, just go for it. Judge how vigorously you move with your baby by her responses: smiling and laughing mean "yes, more"; fussing or crying means "slow down" or "stop." Be creative with your movement. Dance with your baby in your arms, or put the baby down and keep dancing. Ham it up. Your baby is a terrific partner and audience.

Dancing, playing, and singing are essential parts of growing up. Your baby first learns these activities and how to appreciate them from you. Traditionally dance and music originated in the home. Our culture puts them on stage, which is nice, but they belong at home too.

Playing is good exercise. Pretend you are harvesting or hunting. Growl like a lion. Sing out at the top of your lungs or very softly. Two sticks become rhythm instruments. An oatmeal box is your baby's drum. Go ahead, get crazy. Get sweaty. Be a child with your child.

Cool-Down Gravity Roll

Just as you must always warm up before vigorous activity, you must cool down before you stop. Do this gravity roll. Then rub your muscles, stretch and walk around a bit.

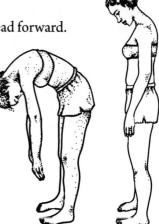

- Stand tall and easy. Drop the weight of your head forward. Take a breath and relax. Feel the pull.

- Let the weight of your head and gravity draw you downward slowly. Breathe. Go as far as you can without straining.

- Hang there. You can make a loud "bbllahh" sound if you like.

- Roll up, one vertebra at a time, beginning at your tailbone.

- You will feel like you are uncurling.

- Let your head come up last.

What About the Blues?

Being 'blue' after having a baby is normal. Your placenta is gone, which accounts for a tremendous drop in serum estrogen and progesterone. Having grown accustomed to heightened levels of pregnancy maintaining hormones coursing through your body, which have now dropped to a fraction of what they were in late pregnancy, you are bound to FEEL the changes.

For many new mothers day three, the day one's milk comes-in, can be particularly emotional. An old midwife's tale says; "The milk flows when the tears flow." So let it flow and Let IT Go! Sadness and elation can come and go at any time. Talking to your midwife, doctor, doula and other mothers can be very soothing.

Favorite Baby Blues Remedies:

- A cup of chamomile or soothing herbal tea, sip it with a friend.
- Warm milk and Honey, with a pinch of cinnamon to soothe & digest.
- Extra rest balanced with gentle activities/exercise.
- A warm bath, spiced with fragrant flowers and/or essential oils
- Plenty of snuggles, kissing and hugging is medicine
- Ask your mother or a trusted aunt to come help, or phone home.
- Ask your mom or a friend to make your favorite food, eat it up!
- Wear blue, Mary the mother of Jesus was said to have done this.
- Start a creative project, simple and fulfilling, that you can do from home.
- Ask your caregiver about homeopathic, herbal or flower remedies.
- Breastfeed often, drinking in your baby as you do it.
- Plant something in the garden.
- Read and write poetry. Sing. Light a candle. Pray
- Feeling brings crying, tears are healing, they wash our souls. The angels weigh each precious tear. Your ups and downs will stabilized as your hormones find their new balance.

Essential oils for banishing baby blues:

- Rose: Helps balance hormones & relieves anxiety, legend says the rose is antidepressant.
- Bergamot ~~ That special fragrance of "earl grey" tea is soothing, fever reducing, antidepressant, analgesic.
- Geranium ~~ Reduces stress, lessens depression, balances hormones, supports kidneys and can reduce high blood pressure.
- Angelica ~~ Antispasmodic for moms suffering painful after-contractions, calms nerves, supports the liver, purifying.
- Mandarin ~~ Relaxes nerves, a gentle sedative, for the new mother who is too tired to sleep. Try a few drops of Mandarin essential oil on your pillow, and sleep when your baby has a late morning and afternoon nap.
- Grapefruit ~~ Reduces sugar cravings and abates fluid retention, stimulates immune system and decreases depression.
- Melissa ~ Helps you to feel you belong on this Earth. Calms nerves, helps you sweat. A tonic that inspires well-being, reduces high blood pressure.

Try these separately or in your favorite combinations in relaxing baths. Remember that essential oils are very concentrated, only a few drops is enough for a full tub. There are also oil infusers for your home. I love the real thing; a bouquet of roses or a nose-gay of geraniums, a bowl of mandarin oranges, a glass of freshly squeezed grapefruit juice. It is becoming easier to find pure essential oils online and in healthy stores.

Essential Oils to Promote Lactation

- Calry Sage – helps the very new mother to bring her milk in, apply diluted with coconut or olive oil, to bottom of your feet.
- Basil & Gernaium – for mother's milk production
- Fennel – brings your milk in, helps to maintain milk production
- Peppermint – helps decrease milk production, in case of engorged breasts.

***Statements about essential oils have not been evaluated by the FDA. These oils are only intended to support mother's well being. They are not intended to treat, diagnose, decrease severity, prevent, or cure any illness, condition or disease.

Postpartum Depression (PPD)

Because childbirth is often a woman's most significant life event, society would have us believe it is a universally happy event. The truth is women are extremely vulnerable psychologically during the first year or more postpartum. Being a new mother is a balance of blues and bliss, if the balance is off postpartum depression may set it.

Postpartum depression (PPD) strikes 10 to 20 percent of new mothers. Unlike the blues PPD does not go away within a few days. Postpartum blues usually begin, the third or forth day postpartum. Postpartum depression's onset typically occurs between day one and six weeks postpartum. However it may not develop right away. Sometimes PPD sets in weeks and even up to eighteen months or more after you've had a baby. Postpartum depression can be insidious and catastrophic. It can last up to a year, even longer. If you have had trauma in your life, and/or trauma associated with your childbirth experience, you may suffer from post traumatic stress disorder (PTSD), in addition to postpartum depression (PPD). It will be important that your family finds you good professional help for coping and healing.

Symptoms of PPD –Few women suffer from all of these, and the severity of the symptoms varies from woman to woman and from day to day:

- Sleepless nights but feeling you could sleep all day
- Sore breasts (not engorged)
- Loss of Appetite
- Nightmares
- Clumsiness
- General exhaustion
- Unquenchable thirst
- Bloating
- Irritability
- Dizziness
- Backaches
- Fears
- Anxiety attacks
- Either over- or under eating
- Shame
- Loneliness
- Deep despondency
- Mood swings
- Confusion
- Complete loss of interest in sex
- Cravings
- Hopelessness and loss of self
- Headaches
- Frequent crying or inability to cry
- Mental incompetence
- Increasing desire for alcoholic beverages, sedatives

Women who tend to get premenstrual syndrome (PMS) will notice that postpartum depression has the same symptoms as PMS. Treatments for PPD and PMS are similar. What differentiates PPD from PMS is the duration of the symptoms. When a woman has PMS, she gets relief between the onset of menstruation and ovulation. The woman who is suffering from postpartum depression has no relief from the discomfort and life-disruption of these symptoms. Yet there seems to be a correlation between getting PMS and having postpartum depression.

Women of all ages, races and lifestyles find themselves immersed in postpartum depression. It is impossible to predict who will suffer from it. Having no symptoms of PPD after your first baby does not guarantee you will not suffer from it following subsequent births. Women who have suffered from PPD following previous births are at greater risk of having it again. If you suffered PPD once and are again pregnant, take time to establish a strong network of support, before the baby is born. Let the people closest to you know just how vulnerable you will be in the postpartum period. Arrange to have at least one responsible and loving adult with you around the clock, for at least the first three weeks following the birth.

Do not be ashamed to seek both loving support and professional help. Postpartum depression is not your fault. It does not mean that you are not a loving, caring mother. PPD is caused by body chemistry and is exacerbated by stress. You could not have chosen this life test. You will need help to get through it, and that's really O.K. Family and friends of a woman who is suffering from PPD, please get involved. Help by finding a health care professional who has had experience with PPD. Don't let this go.

Coping with PPD

Coping is a daily undertaking for women with postpartum depression. It will take courage and determination to get from each sunrise to sunset. The following advice has helped many women through difficult times.

- Be certain to get enough rest.
- Balance rest with healthy activity.
- Don't watch too much T.V. Limit the time you spend on social media and internet.
- Do something special, just for you, everyday. (a nice walk, a massage, a manicure, read a few chapters of a book you love, etc)
- Take a good look at your diet. Are you getting what you need nutritionally? Eliminate caffeine, refined sugars, excess salt and you may find the symptoms of PPD are reduced. Eat three main meals a day and three small meals in between.
- To ward off fatigue you need fuel, keep high-protein snacks on hand.
- Reduce your sweets, but make sure you have comfort foods, feed your body & Soul.
- Eat healthy carbohydrates every day. This is also fuel.
- Avoid isolation. Share the company of a friend or family member EACH day. You may find comfort and support from other women who have also suffered from and survived PPD, seek them out, they want to help you.
- Exercise every day. Dance and stretch, move, walk briskly, swim.
- Relax. Prayer and/or meditation, or yoga are powerful soul-medicine.
- Reduce stress. Breathe deeply, do neck rolls. Try not to worry about small details.
- Read an inspirational book.
- Let some things go: laundry, dirty dishes, ask for help.
- Get out in your flower or vegetable garden, or grow something indoors. Mother Earth will share your pain.

If things get out of hand or you feel even a little unable to cope, **SEEK PROFESSIONAL HELP. PPD is nothing to be ashamed of.**

If you hear voices, or have strange impressions, seek professional help right away. Some postpartum mothers suffer for Psychosis, and this demands you have immediate professional attention from a doctor of psychology, who has experience with PPD and Postpartum Psychosis.

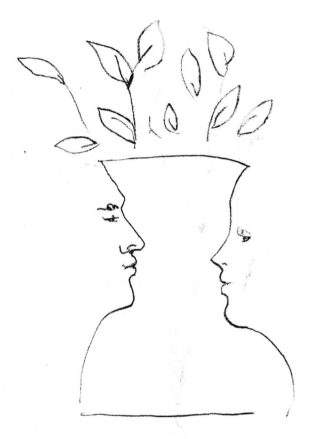

"Sun, moon, stars... You that move in the heavens,
Hear this Mother!
A new life has come among you.
Make it's life smooth."
~ from an Omaha Native American ceremony for
newborn babies

Postpartum Care according to ancient Ayurvedic principles

by Marjan De Jong

The birth of a baby is one of the most beautiful events in the life of a woman. Though, the transition from carrying to caring for a baby can be very challenging for the mother's health; physically and emotionally. To avoid feeling exhausted and overwhelmed Ayurveda offers herbalized oil massages, dietary guidelines, routine advice and herbal preparations, to actively restore the mother's natural balance, strength and stamina. Of course there is also care to create balance in the newborn baby.

Ayurveda, the traditional healthcare system of India, calls the first 6 weeks following delivery "Kaya Kalpa". A period in which there is a lot of focus on the recovery of new mothers and the bonding with the baby. During this period the new mothers are being nourished and taken care off with special meals that are being cooked, postpartum herbal preparations and above all it's been made sure that the new mother takes REST. Rest, rest and more rest. All to actively restore the mother's natural balance, strength and stamina. The principle behind this is, that when you mother the mother, she will have the energy and love to take care of her newborn.

You might be wondering why are these massages, herbal supplements etc. so important. Is just rest not enough. Yes, rest is very important! But to understand the importance of the different aspects of ayurvedic postpartum care, I have to tell you a bit more about Ayurveda.

According to Ayurveda everything in creation composed of 5 basic elements (mahabhutas); space, air, water, fire and earth. These same building blocks form our human body. They are responsible for the 3 metabolic principles, doshas, which govern our body. The principles are: Vata, Pitta and Kapha. Every person is born with its own unique combination of these 3 principles.

Following you see an overview of the doshas, their qualities and functions. This will help you to understand the various aspects of the postpartum care.

Dosha	Elements	Qualities	Bodily Functions
Vata	Space and air	Moving, quick, Light, Cold, rough, dry Leads the other doshas	Concerning movement Controls the activities of the nervous system and the process of elimination
Pitta	Fire	Hot, Sharp, Light, acid, Slightly oily	Concerning metabolism and heat regulation Governs the digestive functions of the body
Kapha	Water and air	Heavy, oily, slow, cold, sweet, steady, sticky and soft	Concerns the structural aspects of the body and is responsible for biological strength, proper body structure

During pregnancy and delivery the natural balance of the mother changes drastically, especially the Vata dosha who is responsible for the process of giving birth. According to Ayurveda, postpartum fatigue, mood swings, constipation, anxiety, and depression are caused by an imbalance in the Vata dosha, which can become aggravated during childbirth. This is the reason that every aspect of the postpartum care is designed to balance the Vata dosha. Vata is the air and space, or wind in our bodies. To maintain pregnancy Vata moves upward within the body. When Labor begins the Vata reverses and moves downward, to support childbirth so the baby may be safely expelled.

Now you have a bit of understanding about the doshas, their qualities and functions, let's talk about the various aspects of Ayurveda that will help to bring the Vata dosha back into balance.

1. Rest!
2. Daily rejuvenating massages with special herbalized oils for the mother in the convenience of her own home. Followed by bed rest and warm bath soak.
3. Herbal supplements to support recovery, digestion & breastfeeding.
4. Dietary guidelines
5. Advices for daily routine.
6. Hands on instruction in baby massage & exercises.

1. Rest ~ Being rather than Doing

This is the most important thing you can do for yourself after your baby has been born. For the coming 6 weeks rest when the baby sleeps. Either by taking a nap, by meditating, getting a massage, having a warm bath. But take your rest. You probably will have the tendency to do things, due to an aggravated Vata, (the wind in your body trying to find it's balance again after childbirth) but resist this and be grateful for all the people who offer help and give you the chance to enjoy quality and quite time with your baby and the rest of your intimate family. And dad please take care that mom settles down, protect her from negative influences and doing instead of being.

2. Arrange for daily massages by a trained Ayurvedic postpartum masseuse

The daily massages with warm herbalized oils followed by a heat treatment, some rest or nap (yes you won't be the first one who falls asleep during or after the massage and find yourself snoring) and a nice warm bath, is such a great boon. You might not feel like getting a massage, but believe me once they start you don't want them to stop.

While massaging a young woman, she started crying. She told me that she was in such a shock after giving birth and that now she started to feel that she was getting whole again. You can imagine that that brought tears to my eyes too.

Another lady who had trouble nursing came running towards me, giving me a huge hug and told me that, after her massage her milk started flowing and that she was done nursing in 10 minutes instead of 1 hour with still a crying baby before.

Getting a massage everyday from an Ayurvedic postpartum masseuse is for most people not feasible, but even 1-2 times a week and giving yourself a massage with warm sesame oil and taking a warm shower or bath on the other days is doing miracles. You will see that the massages provides you with deep rest, increase vitality and stamina, helps to guide your body back in shape, makes lactation easier, increases circulation, tones muscles and calms your nervous system. These are just a few of the benefits.

3.Herbal supplements

Within the vast knowledge of Ayurvedic Medicine there are a couple of herbal recommendation for after given birth. All tailored to reduce Vata, strengthening the digestive system, promoting a healthy flow of breastmilk. I'll mention 2 here

Fennel and fenugreek tea is one of them – known to decrease Vata (air/wind) in the digestive system. It's been recommended to make a tea out of this mixture and to drink throughout the day. When mother drinks this digestive aid tea, it helps keep baby from becoming gassy.

Another favourite is: New Mother's Tea – A kind of strong tea made of 10 different root herbs. Despite its taste, moms just love it. I think we instinctively know just how good this herbal combination is. It helps the body to remove Vata from the tissues, it's very calming, benefits the pelvic organs and pelvic region and it is gently purifying.

4. Dietary guidelines

After giving birth the digestive fire, called Agni, is often diminished, making the mothers' digestion as tender as the baby's. These guidelines are designed so that the food is easy digestible and at the same strengthens the digestive fire.

How well your food is digested, and what kind of food you eat determines the quality of your milk and the well being of your baby, and, your own well being too.

In nutshell you can say that food should be fresh, very simple, wholesome, consisting of warm, liquid and unctuous organic foods that are of the sweet, sour and salty taste categories... and cooked with love.

Foods to favour:

- **Dairy:** Whole organic milk (unless you are milk intolerant)
- **Sweeteners:** Molasses, raw sugar, succanat, and honey (don't heat over 40 Celsius/104 F)
- **Oils:** Ghee (clarified butter), sesame oil, olive oil

- **Grains & Staple foods:** Basmati Rice (white) cook with extra cup of water per cup of rice, unleavened wheat (with Ghee), yams, sweet potatoes, winter squashes oats and quinoa in smaller quantity

- **Fruit:** Favour sweet, ripe fruits like sweet apple, avocado, berries, cherries coconut, currants, dates, figs, grapes, mango, papaya, peaches, raisins, sweet pineapple, plums (soak dried fruits first)

- **Vegetables:** artichoke, asparagus, beet, carrots, cucumber, (peeled) eggplant, yellow squash, butternut squash, and acorn squash, pumpkin, and zucchini. After 2 weeks you can add spinach and green beans.

- **Protein:** boiled milk, sesame and almond milk, unfermented cheeses (after 2 weeks), yellow split mung dahl, tofu (after 4th week)

- **Seasonings:** basil, black pepper (limited), brown mustard seeds, caraway, cardamom, cinnamon, cumin, fennel, fenugreek, ginger, lime or lemon juice, marjoram, paprika, saffron, salt (after first few days), tamarind, and turmeric.

- **Nuts:** Blanched almonds, finely ground

- **Meat:** Try to avoid eating meat in the first month after delivery. You can make a broth from organic chicken, turkey or fish.

Be careful with the following vegetables even after the 6 weeks period as long as you are nursing: broccoli, cauliflower, cabbage, chillies garlic, brussel sprouts, potatoes, kale, green peas, green pepper, onions, sprouts and in general raw vegetable (salads). These foods are hard to digest and known to cause gas. And please be nice to yourself and avoid coffee, sodas, chocolate, alcohol, frozen or microwave foods and leftovers!!!

For those who are going to be the "chef cook", I would say be as creative as you want with these guidelines, give it your own signature. And cook with LOVE, this is the most important ingredient! Keep in mind to start with very easy digestible, soupy like foods. Just to give you an idea for the first days. Mothers often say that they prefer eating warm vegetable soups or creamy breakfast cereals. To get some more ideas, I have added a few recipes.

First meal: A good first meal that can even be prepared during labour is Konji; a type of rice porridge. To make this, bring 16 cups (3,8 liter) of water to a boil. Add 1 cup (±200g) basmati rice and a bit of ghee. Bring to a boil and let simmer without a lid for several hours, stirring occasionally. In the end add a generous amount of iron rich sugar (i.e. succanat), saffron and some powdered ginger, black pepper, cinnamon and cardamom to it aid digestion. Serve this dish throughout the day with ghee and extra sugar.

Some mother's prefer a savoury soup, this rice Konji can be flavoured after cooking is finished, with miso, instead of sugar. But anyway the first dish should be very easy to digest

Vegetable soup, use any combination of vegetables from the "foods to favour " list. Very nice to serve with chapattis (unleavened Indian breads).

- 6 cups (±1,5 l.) of water
- 4 cups (950 ml) chopped vegetables
- 1 teaspoon salt or use a vegetable broth without yeast to taste
- 1 tablespoon ghee
- 1 teaspoon brown mustard seeds
- ½ teaspoon of ground cumin
- ½ teaspoon of ground fenugreek
- some fresh shredded ginger

Melt the ghee in a large pot. Add the mustard seeds, when they start dancing add the other spices, sauté for 1 minute. Add the mixed, washed vegetables and sauté for another 5-10 minutes over low heat. Add boiling water with salt or your stock and let's simmer for 30 minutes.

Khichari is a traditional Indian dish made by thoroughly cooking rice and dahl together. It is very nourishing and easy to digest. (Serves 2-3)

- ⅓ cup (100 g) mung lentils (cleaned and washed)
- ½ cup (100 g) basmati rice
- 2½ cups (600 ml) water
- 2 tablespoons ghee
- 1 tablespoon freshly minced ginger
- 1 teaspoon cumin seeds
- 1 teaspoon black mustard seeds
- 1 teaspoon salt
- ¼ teaspoon saffron (optional)

Bring the rice, beans and water to a boil and let them simmer until the dahl is tender and all the water is absorbed. This takes about 1 ½ hour. Stir occasionally so the mixture doesn't stick to bottom of the pot, and add some more water if necessary. The khichari should have the consistency of thick gravy. When the dahl and rice are ready, heat the ghee in a small skillet. Add the fresh ginger mustard, cumin and fenugreek seeds. Sautee them over low heat till you hear the mustard seeds "dance". Add to the khichari. Stir in the turmeric and salt and serve.

Delicious yams. Moms love them and they are vey easy to prepare. Bake, boil or steam the yams till they are tender. Mash them, add ghee and some nice spices like cinnamon, cardamom, ginger a bit of salt, and if you feel like a bit of cream. If you like to surprise the children too, make "French fries" out of them. Simply peel and cut the yams, sprinkle them with some salt and olive oil and bake them in the oven. It's just delicious.

Warm fruits compote. Stew fruits from the list with a cinnamon stick, some cloves, cardamom, anise and some ginger. If needed add some raw sugar. A pinch of salt, to enhance the taste, can be added after the first days.

Almond snack. Mix 4-5 blanched almonds, a handful of raisins or some dates, and two teaspoons of grated coconut. Or you can blend a batch in a food processor and make small balls.

Rice pudding. This can be made as a meal or a snack. (serves 3-4)
- ½ cup (100 g) white basmati rice
- few saffron threads
- 4 cups (950 ml) milk or milk replacement (like almond milk)
- ½ cup (100 g) raw sugar
- pinch of cardamom
- rosewater
- chopped soaked blanched almonds

Mix softly boiled basmati rice with raisins, raw sugar, cardamom, cinnamon, blanched almonds and or saffron. Cover the mixture with milk or almond milk and bake it in the oven till all the milk is

Easy fresh rice milk (recipe from Ysha Oakes a cooked variation with added ghee for postpartum) This milk can be served after childbirth. (serves 3-4)
- ⅓ cup (70 g) basmati rice or brown basmati rice
- 3 cups (710 ml) water
- ½ stick cinnamon
- 1-2 whole cloves
- 2 pinches salt
- ½ teaspoon vanilla
- 4 teaspoons ghee, sesame or sunflower oil
- to taste add raw sugar or agave

Soak the rice, cinnamon stick and cloves overnight in 1 cup (250 ml) water. Drain and rinse. Combine the rice and the boiling water and cinnamon in a blender till smooth. Strain if desired. Bring the rice milk to a boil over medium heat, stirring constantly. When boiled it is done. Add the salt, vanilla, ghee or oil and sugar to taste. Serve hot with a teaspoon of extra ghee.

Almond-date shake. This shake was one of my favourite shakes that I continued to use just because it tasted so good and is so nourishing especially when you are nursing and you can use an extra boost. It can be served a week or so after giving birth.

- 10 medium, pitted and soaked dates (or 3-4 of these divine medjool dates, no soaking needed)
- ½ cup (70 g) soaked blanched almonds
- 2 cups (± 500ml) warm water for making the milk
- a pinch of cardamom and ginger
- a few threads of saffron

Soak the pitted dates and almonds in separate bowls overnight. Drain and peel the almonds. Blend with fresh water until smooth. If the consistency is too thick, just add some water. The ginger and cardamom help with the digestion of the almonds.

Lassi is an excellent digestive aid and can be taken during or after meals. It is best made of fresh, homemade yoghurt.

- 1 cup (±250 ml) yoghurt
- 2-5 cups (±0,5-1,2l) water
- a pinch of cardamom
- 3 tablespoons sugar or honey
- a few drops of rosewater (optional)

Mix ingredients well. There are many variations on lassi. A favourite is mango lassi. Very simple. Just add a peeled mango to the ingredient and enjoy!

And last but not least, let me tell you how to make ghee, since this is very important in balancing Vata and has been mentioned in more than one recipe.

Ghee. Making ghee is not difficult. Ghee is made by simmering butter until the water evaporates and solids separate from the oil. The easiest way to make ghee is by using a crockpot. Though you have the freedom to leave, make sure to check in now and then to see how the process is going.

2 pounds (900 g) of organic unsalted butter will makes about 1½ pounds (675 g) ghee.

Place the butter in your pot on low setting. Start early in the morning and let it cook all day uncovered, very gently. Most solids will sink to the bottom, but some will stay on top. They will brown which adds to the flavour of the ghee. Be careful though that they don't burn. The ghee is ready when there is a white or golden crust on top, or the white sediments start to turn brown.

Skim the crust from the top, and poor the ghee through a sieve lined with a cotton cloth in a glass jar. Keep it closed and stored in a dark place.

You can also make ghee on the stove. Just choose the heaviest pot you have and melt the butter over low heat. Placing a heat diffuser on the burner is helpful.

5. Daily Postpartum Routine

There are a lot of things that could be said, but I like to keep it simple here. Rest whenever you can, enjoy each other and the baby, and let people take care of you

Try waking up early in the morning and going to bed on time in the eve before 10PM. Avoid watching TV at night since it aggravates Vata. In the morning get a massage or massage yourself in the morning. After you have eaten, massage and nurse the baby. Drink when the baby drinks and be as regular as you can with your meals with the main meal of the day around noon. ENJOY the baby and each other. Let someone else take care of household duties. This is your "Baby~Moon" savor each moment.

Enjoy the comfort of your home in the first 6 weeks. After 2 weeks you can go for a small stroll if you feel like. Go around in your yard or in another quiet place, but avoid shopping malls for now, also avoid places with harsh lights or loud sounds. And don't go out on very windy or cold days. If you have to, make sure to cover your head and the baby's head. Since Vata gets easily aggravated because of wind and that's the last thing we would like. Actually Ayurveda suggest having the baby wear a hat/ cap for the first year. The fontanel is not closed yet and it is a way to protect the tender nervous system of the new born.

A special note about visiting hours. I can imagine that you burst of proud and can't wait to introduce your baby to relatives and friends, and they are anxiously waiting to see your new family member! Try to make these visits short, or organize a Welcome party after the first 6 weeks. Always ask visitors to wash their hands, before touching your new baby.

6. Baby massage

> *"The best life insurance for your baby is a daily massage*
> *and mother's milk"* ~ *Dr. S Gogte*

About 10-12 days after the delivery, or as soon as the umbilical cord has come off and the wound is well healed, you may learn/ start the baby massaging your baby. You can do it twice a day, one time in the morning before drawing a bath, and a short version in the evening followed by nursing and then sleep. In the evening use less oil and no bath. The oil brings calmness to the nervous system, and you will see that your baby will have a sound sleep.

Massaging your newborn is not just pure joy, the massage improves your baby's digestion, tones the muscles, enhances relaxation and establishes better sleeping patterns. Giving Baby a massage is a way to bond, especially for the dads. I remember several times when I was massaging a mother while the baby was receiving a massage from the dad.

Before beginning a massage, make sure baby has breastfed well, and is settled. Turn off your phone, this is a time of peace and quiet.

You may wish to have someone play or put on gentle music. Make sure the room is war enough for baby to be comfortable while naked. It the very warm months massaging baby outdoors is wonderful, make sure there is no wind. Avoid direct hot sun, as it can burn baby's skin and harm his or her eyes.

It's always so nice to see how the baby's enjoy and relax. And yes, you have to be prepared because relaxation often goes hand in hand with peeing and/or pooping, and that can give hilarious situations if you're not prepared.

Use only a pure, unscented, certified organic oils. Do not use mineral oil on your baby's skin, nor your skin. Fragrances are not necessary and may be too harsh. Never put essential oils directly on baby's skin. Diffusing a calming essential oil into the environment is very nice.

You may use these oils, or a blend of them:

- Virgin Coconut oil reduces fire for the baby who gets red rashes, or has a bit of hot temperament.
- Sweet Almond oil may promote the health of baby's skin.
- Sesame oil nourishes and warms the baby's body.

1. Place the oil in a squeeze bottle and slightly warm the oil by placing the squeeze bottle in a pot of hot water. Keep a small to medium sized towel nearby, to wipe excess oil from your hands, as needed.

2. Draw a warm bath into a baby bathtub, and make ready, right beside where you will be doing the massage. Massage baby on the floor, so there is no risk of baby slipping and falling. I lay out yoga mats, and place old towels on them, for my comfort and baby's safety.

3. In a warm room, on or a sunny porch with no wind, put a towel on your lap. Place your undressed baby facing up in your lap. If comfortable, you can use the traditional method of sitting with legs straight out and the baby supported on your legs. You may wish to put your back against a wall, for support.

4. After testing the temperature of the oil, take some oil in both hands and apply to the baby's scalp. Gently make little circles all over the baby's scalp. Be very gentle, as the baby still has a soft spot in the skull.

5. Move down to the arms. Take more oil for each step as needed. Massage by moving down and then up each arm, using long strokes for the long bones, and circular strokes on the joints. Massage the palms and each of baby's fingers. Never be too harsh, gentle but firm pressure is good. Find a resonance with your fingers and hands, soothing the baby's body and spirit.

6. Take more oil as needed, and repeat this gentle but firm process for the legs. Remember you are stimulating baby's circulation but calming his or her spirit. Use soothing strokes and intention.

7. Now make circles over baby's chest and gently follow along the collar bones. Next massage baby's abdomen in large clockwise circles, following the direction that bowel movements flow. Don't be surprised if baby passes gas or even has a BM.

8. Carefully, using the nearby small towel to prevent baby from slipping, turn the baby over onto his or her belly, and massage baby's back and buttocks. Use long strokes on baby's back and flanks, and circular strokes on the buttocks.

9. Again, using the towel to prevent slipping, turn baby back over to finish on the face, again with gentle strokes. . Make upward strokes on baby's third eye, then small circles, on baby's face, massaging cheeks, forehead, chin, ears, stroking neck and jaws. Massage along the nose, above the nose, and along the chin.

10. Now check temperature of the bath you have already made ready. You may lower baby, and the towel he or she has been laying on, right into the water. The towel, or a cotton baby blanket will guard against slipping. No need to use soap. If you do wish to have some mild cleansing suds, simply grind a hand full of instant oatmeal in your blender. This makes a cleansing, soothing bath powser. Let the warm water dilute the healthy oil. Babies love to play and express pleasure in the bath, have some fun.

11. Wrap your baby snuggly in a towel. Now the baby is usually ready for a good nap and some sweet dreaming. The father of my children made massaging our babies a daily routine. Once they became toddlers, they would sometimes get bored and wiggle away. Be flexible and enjoy Baby Massage. If your day has been too full, and an oil massage is not possible, massage your baby right through her or his clothing, whenever you are holding and hugging and hanging out.

Having read all, you might think now what can I do, how can apply this knowledge? The answer is: Make a postpartum plan!

Just as you have been preparing for your Birth, prepare for the period when the baby has arrived. Make your wishes known. Maybe during your baby shower or another occasion and see who would like to help or contribute towards the massages. I can't think of a better gift to give.

Food Train for the Family

It is very special if the new mother's best friend, or a sister can create a list, or a Food Train, for people who would like to cook for the postpartum family during the first few weeks after Baby's arrival. Make sure there are back ups meal providers as well. Volunteers can fill in the Food Train list, requesting days they can conveniently cook. The organizer should provide the volunteer cooks with some dietary guidelines/recipes, like the ones suggested in this book. Volunteers should plan to make the main, midday meal, providing enough food for the Mother, her partner and any other children in the family. I like to provide some extra dishes, so there is plenty for mother to snack later.

I have had the luxury that both times when I gave birth to my girls, I was living in a community were there was something set up. Whenever someone was pregnant, a list was going around of who was going to cook when. It was wonderful receiving the trays with special prepared foods, often accompanied with a beautiful card or something else. Everyone liked to be part of the Food Train. 1. The cooks were able to see the new baby and 2. They knew that when they were pregnant something would be organized for them as well.

But maybe your partner is a great cook and likes to take this responsibility or another relative or good friend. I have also massaged a lady who had hired someone to cook for her food.

Think together with your husband/ partner and sisters/friends how you would like your postpartum period to be. Make a plan so that the only thing you have to think of after giving birth, is the baby, and taking time to rest and recover.

What to think about when planning for Baby~Moon

Ask for help from your Sisters/Friends, when planning your postpartum Baby-Moon. Some practical suggestions: stock up on dry foods like rice and dahl, herbs and spices, making a grocery list, see if there are friends who would like to help with household duties, taking care of the children, cooking or whatever you feel that would help you. And believe me, this sounds easier than done. It might be so tempting to run an errand, do the laundry, etc. With Vata being up and swirling to your body it might be harder than you think to give in and enjoy this special Baby~Moon time.

Good luck and enjoy. Have a wonderful birth and embrace the postpartum period with Love and Rest.

LAM – Nature's Own Child Spacing...

Breastfeeding suppresses fertility. This is called, Lactation Amenorrhea Method or LAM. To be a dependable method of child spacing, the following three criteria must be met:

- Your menstrual cycles have NOT returned.
- Your Baby is fully exclusively breastfeeding – no water, no supplements, no rubber nipples or dummies.
- Your Baby is less than six months old.

Only between .5 and 3 women in 100 per year get pregnant while following these guidelines for LAM. All three guidelines must be met or your chances of unintended pregnancy are greater.

Natural Family Planning: Billings Ovulation Method

Natural Family Planning (NFP) is completely possible. This technique of family planning is very effective, it is not Rhythm Method, and it is scientifically proven. Rhythm Method is NOT Family Planning, it planning a big family!

Using NFP effectively, takes commitment from both the man and the woman. Communication is also essential, for the method to work. The woman must observe her symptoms of possible fertility every day, all day, and she must keep a chart of these symptoms.

Woman: "Am I wet or is my vulva dry?"

Both partners must communicate, and either the man or the woman may mark the chart.

Woman: "Honey, today I observed wetness."

Man: "OK, I'll mark that on our NFP chart by the bed."

Last step: follow the simple rules!

Woman: "Honey, you know this means we must abstain from lovemaking for as long as I have wetness, as I am most likely ovulating. Unless, you're ready to have another baby. "

Man: "Well dear, let's wait and enjoy the wee baby we already have. Remember, we must also abstain for 3 days of dryness, after all wetness has gone. No worries Sweetie, I'm planning a honeymoon for us, as soon as we have the green light for lovemaking again!"

For COMPLETE information, and instruction in NFP see this website:

billings.life

learnnfponline.com/billings-ovulation-method

The rewards are many: The woman need not poison herself or risk her health with artificial methods of birth control. Harming the mother, to control population is violence. We observe that couples who fully commit to NFP, which is truly a lifestyle of non-violence, fall more deeply in love.

Making Your Own Postpartum Moon Pads

"What a hassle." Might be your first thought when we suggest you make your own personal moon (menstrual) pads. Think about it a minute. Ask yourself two questions; "Are commercial pads environmentally wise?" "Are the commercial pads made with my health in mind?"

The answer to the first question is: No, commercial pads are not kind to our environment. They end up in landfills. This poses a threat to the public health. Some brands claim to be made consciously with organic cotton, I would choose these, if going for "disposable" pads.

As for the answer to the second question, sadly it too is; "No, most commercially manufactured menstrual pads and tampons are not healthy for women's bodies. Most brands of pads and tampons contain two potentially harmful components, rayon (for absorbency) and dioxin (a chemical used to bleach the products). Dioxin is potentially cancer-associated, it can break down your immune system, harm your reproductive system and cause endometriosis. In men it is associated with lower sperm counts. The rayon in tampons is so absorbent that when the tampon is removed, rayon fibers are left behind. This serves as a breeding ground for bacteria.

The use of tampons, especially the 'high-absorbency' kind, put women at risk for contracting toxic shock syndrome (TSS). For this reason I advise all women, of all ages, against the use of tampons. TSS is a potentially life-threatening systemic disorder. The symptoms are, fever of sudden onset, Hypotension (low-blood pressure) and rash (most prominent on the palms and soles of feet). Toxic shock syndrome is acute for 4 to 5 days, there is a 1 to 2 week convalescent phase.

There are alternative companies who manufacture organic cotton tampons and pads that are unbleached. If you are going to buy pads, buy only these. Why take chances with your health, while the manufactures of these products make a profit?

We found making our own pads to be a fun activity. Women may enjoy gathering for an old fashioned sewing circle. Together you can share stories, sip tea and make moon pads, which are both healthy and Mother Earth friendly.

Soak your Moon Pads in water, after using them. then, pour this water, rich with the minerals and stem cells of your menstrual blood, into the Earth Mother. Water a tree or your garden with it. You will be amazed at the growth.

What you need to make 6-7 moon pads:

- 1½ yards of soft 100% cotton flannel or bird's eye cotton (there are no rules saying your moon pads must be all white, let yourself go, choose some fun prints and colors).
- A pair of sharp scissors.
- 6 or more medium size sew-on snaps.
- Thread for sewing.
- You may use a sewing machine. It is also fun to hand stitch our moon pads with brightly colored embroidery threads.

MID PANEL

Cut 6 pieces of this pattern for each pad

1. Layer all 6 pieces together.
2. Along both sides insert the wing piece ¼ inch, between the third and fourth layers. Baste or secure with pins.
3. Use the zigzag setting on your sewing machine, or blanket stitch all along all edges.
4. Secure all six layers of cloth together with the wings protruding evenly from the sides.
5. Next add the snap, which will hold your moon pad securely folded around the narrow part of your underpants.
6. By folding the wings under the mid panel, you can see how the snaps should be sewn on. The 'male' snap portion on one side and the 'female' on the other, so that once in place the moon pad hugs your panty and fits snugly and flat.

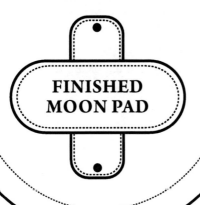

FINISHED MOON PAD

WING PIECE

Cut 2 pieces of this pattern for each pad

1. Fold 1 wing piece in half with the 'right side' inside.
2. Stitch together along the curved edge, leaving a 1 inch section open.
3. Turn right-side-out and close the open section.
4. you may now make decorative stitches along the curved edge.
5. Do the same as above using the other wing piece.

Earth Friendly Diapers

The only truly Earth friendly diapers are those made of cloth, which you wash and reuse. The "disposable" diapers that are sold, are not at all disposable. Even the ones that advertise being biodegradable, have been found not to be. Most of the single use paper and plastic diapers contain chemicals and substances to reduce odor, make them white, and make them extra absorbent, these substances are not healthy for your baby. The skin is an organ; we would not soak our babies' heart or lungs in potentially harmful substances. Why would we take this risk with our babies' skin?

When washing cloth diapers, use soap that is mild and natural. Be sure to double rinse out all soap residue. Drying the diapers in the sun sterilizes them and keeps them super fresh.

There are many wonderful diaper covers on the market. Even if you cringe at the price, they are far less expensive than single use diapers, over time.

Averaging over two years of diaper use per baby, imagine how many trees can be saved, if every natural mother chose Earth friendly cloth diapers. Do it for the Planet, and do it for your Baby.

Some single-use allegedly disposable (but not really disposable) companies try to justify the use of their product, saying that cloth diapers are not environmental because we need to use water to wash them. That's just propaganda, protecting their profits. The water and natural soap you use to wash cloth diapers has much less negative impact on the ecology of our Earth, than diapers made of plastic and trees, or plant fibers, laced with chemicals and bleach. For a healthier baby and to protect our Earth … commit to cloth diapering.

"My mother and father took me in and provided
everything for me - the love, nurturing, basic necessities
- to give me the space to grow wings, so that when I went
out into the world, I could fly."

~ Michael Franti

Beauty and Motherhood

What is more beautiful than a pregnant or breastfeeding woman? New Motherhood is a time of body changes and hormonal fluctuations. You may feel radiant one day and unattractive the next. Be assured that this is a special time, in which you are in direct partnership with the Creator of the Universe, you are in a real way quite divine.

Choosing comfortable natural clothing that fits you well will help you feel beautiful. If you wear make-up, look for natural products and keep it simple. Your natural beauty will shine forth if you are modest and clean. There is no beauty device better than a nice shower and shampoo for your hair. Hair dyes are poisonous and should be avoided by pregnant and breastfeeding mothers.

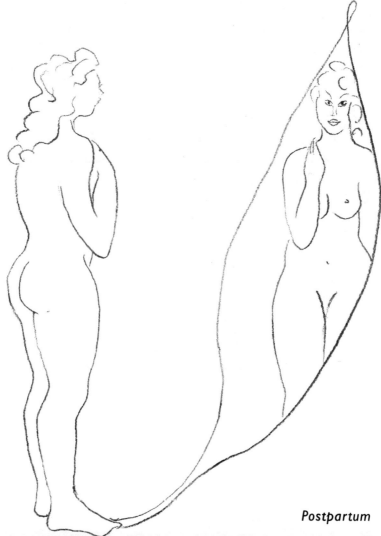

Dress according to your culture. There are many lovely creative ways to wear a krudung or dress for temple or church. At home, let yourself go. Don't be ashamed to be comfortable and to look pretty.

Eating naturally and well is important for maintaining optimal beauty. Please don't diet while pregnant and breastfeeding. Drink plenty of pure water, being well-hydrated makes us more beautiful. Women who enjoy fresh fruits and vegetables really do glow and are naturally lovely.

Rest is nature's least expensive cosmetic. A well-rested woman is beautiful! Reducing stress is a wonderful way to achieve your full loveliness. Meditation, sholate, prayer, a walk in the woods, a nice massage, a relaxing bath scented with essential oils, are all wonderful stress reducers.

Getting some gentle exercise will bring out your beauty as well. Nice walks, swimming, bicycle riding, dancing, etc. all make you feel and look healthier.

A woman in harmony with her spirit is like a river flowing. She goes where she will without pretense and arrives at her destination, prepared to be herself and only herself.

~ Maya Angelou

Living with Baby

Living Organically on our Earth

Becoming a Mother is a true Awakening. Your heart has been stretched and broken open. You now have the "Mommy Brain" that helps you think in a more open way, seeing and evaluating all angles and possibilities. This is as Mother Nature intended it. With the arrival of each baby, you become more loving, more observant and more intelligent. This helps you protect your children, and insures the survival of our species.

Likely, as your pregnancy expands, or soon after your baby arrives in your arms, you will be looking around at your environment, seeing where you can be more Ecological. Don't compromise; make some healthy changes.

Here are some simple household tips to help you make your home more Baby Friendly and MotherEarth Friendly too.

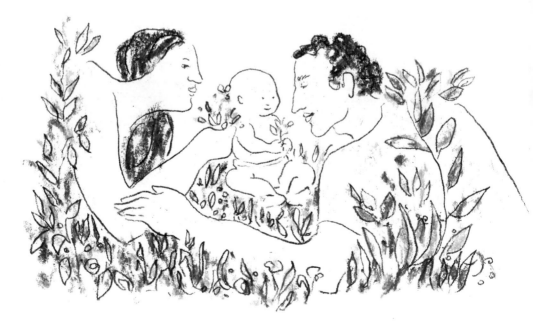

Laundry Soap

Imagine… simply washing your family's clothing and baby's diapers involves profound ecological and health choices!

Most conventional detergents contain toxic chemicals! Including:

- **Fragrance**
- **Surfactants** (which are chemicals like quaternium-15 known to release formaldehyde - a known carcinogen), Diethanolamine (linked with skin and eye irritation and possibly liver problems), Nonlphenol Ethoxylate or NPE (toxic to nerves, irritating to skin, a potential hormone disruptor, toxic to water plants and animals), Linear Alkyl Benzene Sulfonates or LAS (irritating to skin and eyes, and toxic to aquatic life. Benzene on its own is a carcinogen, and when combined with petroleum distillates, is linked to cancer and lung damage)
- STABILIZERS (which includes Polyalkylene Oxide or Ethylene Oxide, linked to eye and lung irritation, and even dermatitis)
- BLEACH (known to irritate skin, eyes, and lungs, and when it mixes with wastewater, can form toxic organic compounds that have been linked with respiratory issues, liver, and kidney damage), Dioxane (causes cancer in mammals and penetrates human skin)
- BRIGHTENERS (like Naphthotriazolystilbenes, linked with developmental and reproductive problems), Benzoxazolyl, Diaminostilbene Disulfonate, Phosphates (associated with environmental damage, particularly in our streams and waterways and causes algae blooms that damage ecosystems), Ethylene Diamine Tetraacetic Acid or EDTA (toxic to animals and is not biodegradable)

Natural Alternatives:

In many places in our world today, a mother can go to a health food store or shop on line for natural and organic soaps for body, laundry and natural household cleaning, as well as other safe and natural body/hygiene products. However, making your own is more economical and there will be no doubt in your mind that it is natural.

Imagine how precious each piece of clothing was when people, mostly girls and women, made each piece by hand. The process was long and elaborate: first growing cotton or other plants or animals to obtain the fibrous materials, next carding the wool or cotton, spinning the threads, weaving the cloth, dyeing for colors, tailoring for clothing. My goodness, you would not just throw a garment that required so much work, into a washing machine with chemical detergent!

Homemade laundry soap:

Soapnuts called Klerek in Indonesia, also called Soapberries: the leathery skinned fruit of the Sapindus tree (from the Lychee family, it grows commonly in warm climates). For centuries people have been using klerek to wash their laundry. In Indonesia, where it is traditionally the soap of choice for fine batik, soapnuts are easy to find. Online, or in Natural Food stores, you may find the Soapnuts or concentrated Soapnut liquid for sale.

How to wash laundry with Soapnuts:

Simply put four to six soapnuts in a small cotton drawstring bag. Pull the string, tightly closing the bag. You can use this bag of soapnuts 7 or more times. If your soapnuts still feel slippery when wet, they are still good. Place the bag of soapnuts with your laundry into the washing machine and wash as usual. Do not overload the machine.

If you are like our family and your laundry is heavily soiled, simply add ¼ cup of baking soda to the machine while the water is filling up.

Separate your whites. If they are stained you may wish to add some lemon juice, as a natural whitener. Remember, sun drying your clothing helps fade away the stains.

After the washing machine is finished with all cycles, simply take out your bag of soapnuts and let it dry.

Hand washing clothing with soapnuts is easy. Soak your bag of soapnuts in a pot of hot water to make a washing "tea" and pour this into your hand washing laundry bucket, mix in ¼ cup of baking soda... and off you go.

Making liquid concentrate laundry soap with Soapnuts:

- ¼ kilo soapnuts
- 1 liter water

Bring soapnuts and water to a boil in a large pot, lower the flame. Simmer until the liquid is reduced to ½. Allow to cool. Store soapnut liquid concentrate in an unbreakable bottle (recycled shampoo bottles work well). To wash clothing, simply add 1/8 cup or a nice squirt for a small to medium load of laundry. For heavily soiled laundry, add ¼ cup of baking soda. This liquid soapnut concentrate is convenient to use when machine or hand washing laundry.

Sodium Bicarbonate also called Baking Soda: It's used in cooking, so it is safe for laundry. Baking soda is mildly disinfectant; it removes odors, makes laundry feel softer, controls fungus, and can be added to any homemade laundry soap. It is used as a leavening to help cakes and other baked goods rise. Since it is edible we know it is safe to wash with.

Other Healthy uses of baking soda for health and hygiene:

Floor wash: Add ¼ cup baking soda to a bucket of warm water, with 1/8 cup vinegar and a few drops of lavender or tea tree essential oil (or a mix of any essential oils you love. Lemon oil is amazing!). Mop your floor with this all-natural cleaner.

Deodorant: Keep baking soda in a small container in your bathroom. After showering, dry off and apply a pinch of the white baking soda under your arms. It is antibacterial, so it prevents odor causing germs from growing on your body, abating bad body odor.

Tooth powder: You may wish to try brushing your teeth with this mildly abrasive powder for it removes plaque. Baking soda is antibacterial, so it reduces tooth decay and keeps gums healthy. It also helps whiten your teeth. Do not use baking soda as a tooth cleaner more than once per week, as the abrasive quality may damage tooth enamel if used too often.

Insect bites: Simply make a paste with 1 tsp. baking soda and enough water to mix into a thick paste. Rub this on mosquito or other bug bites, to neutralize the itching.

Exfoliate your skin: Make a paste by mixing 3 parts baking soda with 1 part water; add a few drops of your favorite essential oil. Rub this briskly onto your skin. Feel the softness when you rinse it off.

Soak your bones: Put ½ cup baking soda, ¹/₈ cup apple cider vinegar and a few drops of your favorite essential oil into a warm bath and soak away stress. This mixture also makes a good footbath.

After sunburn: ½ cup of baking soda in a not-too-warm bath will bring natural relief. Be careful not to towel off too briskly, for your skin may be delicate after too much sun.

Scrubbing paste: Make a paste with 1 cup of baking soda and enough water to form a thick paste, you may add a nice essential oil for fragrance if you like. Keep in a handy jar and use it to scrub pots and pans, clean sinks, countertops, bathtubs and showers, also to disinfect the toilet.

Oatmeal Bath

Oatmeal has been used for centuries to soothe skin, abate rash and treat eczema.

Simply powder 1 cup of oatmeal in a blender, until it is a very fine. Draw a warm bath for baby and wet ½ a handful of the oatmeal powder, smooth this over baby's skin, rinse away after a while. For babies, use this pure, without fragrance. For adults, you may wish to just swirl a generous handful into your warm tub, and add a few drops of jasmine or rose oil along with some rose petals. For dogs with skin problems, wash them with this same oatmeal powder, adding some tea tree oil.

Yoni Toners

Yoni is the word I most prefer to use when referring to our vaginas. Kegel exercises to tighten our yoni's has become controversial, because many women experience too much tightness in their anal sphincter, as a result of too much kegel exercise, and they may become constipated.

Toning your yoni, will enhance all aspects of your health and improve sexual enjoyment by increasing pelvic blood circulation. It is best to learn to love and tone your yoni earlier in life, when one first awakens as a woman. However most women seem to find out about this during pregnancy or in the postpartum period, or after they have problems, like urinary incontinence.

To simply learn yoni toning, try stopping and starting your flow of urine, on the toilet. Toning is NOT only about tightening, it is about letting go. Make sure after trying this on the toilet, you allow all of your urine to finish passing out.

Gently tighten the muscles of your yoni, not your butt or your anus, your yoni... release, tighten again. Each closing/tightening must be followed by an opening/releasing. You may do this quickly and then try doing it slowly. Think of bringing a beam of light up an elevator inside your yoni, now, ever so slowly, release that light down the elevator shaft.

While breastfeeding your baby, or waiting in traffic, is a great time to practice your yoni toners. You can also practice while making love, your partner will let you know how it feels.

Massaging your own belly, is an important way of loving your body and feeling for and finding the strength of your yoni. You will find this also combats constipation while correcting urinary incontinence.

Remember, your pelvic floor holds up all of your organs. Your organ integrity depends upon the strength and suppleness of your pelvic floor. Hold and let go... hold and let go.

Sexuality

If there is no bleeding or excessive cramping love making during pregnancy is safe, and recommended. As your belly grows you will find creative love-making positions. If your partner is male, his semen will help your cervix become ready for childbirth. This is because semen has prostaglandin. This prostaglandin softens your cervix and is absorbed into your body, entering your circulation, where it reaches the baby. This is super good, as prostaglandin helps support healthy fetal brain growth, especially in the 2nd trimester of pregnancy.

After the Baby's birth it is respected in most traditions to wait about 42 days before resuming full sexual relations with your husband. That is not to say that you cannot snuggle and be sensual together.

Your baby naturally sleeps a lot, and this leaves plenty of time for new parents to enjoy their sexuality.

Communicate together about your changing sexuality now that you have become parents. Once you decide you are ready to resume intercourse, talk about it. Make a promise to take it slowly and to stop if there is discomfort. Aim to please each other. Remember sex is a sacred gift. It is the secret that brought your beautiful baby to Earth. It is like a special glue that bonds your marriage and keeps you special for each other.

Sex is a gift from the Divine Creator. It is to be respected and en-JOY-ed.

If your baby dies...

"The woman conceives. As a mother she is another person than the woman without child. She carries the fruit of the night for nine months in her body. Something grows. Something grows into her life that never again departs from it. She is a mother. She is and remains a mother even though her child dies. For at one time she carried the child under her heart. And it does not go out of her heart ever again. Not even when it is dead."

Kore... an Ethiopian woman

The loss of a child is so painful I cannot even articulate here my own fears, my own pain. But something begs to be expressed. Where we live in Indonesia and in the Philippines, many, many women have endured the loss of a child. All over the world, mothers and their families, have lost children. It is difficult to find an extended family that has not lost babies. These mothers are the real heroines of the world. They are the wisest and the finest.

There is no medicine for the pain of losing a baby or a child. Father Time does mend the heart, so that we mothers may carry on, yet life is never the same. Our bodies mend, after the birth-death, but our feelings of love and longing remain. Perhaps this is why women are so exquisitely strong and yet tender.

If you have lost your pregnancy through miscarriage, you have lost a baby. If you have birthed a baby that has died, your empty arms may ache. Only LOVE heals these wounds, and LOVE has many faces. Nothing takes away the scars, they are like the footprints of your baby, tattooed on your soul.

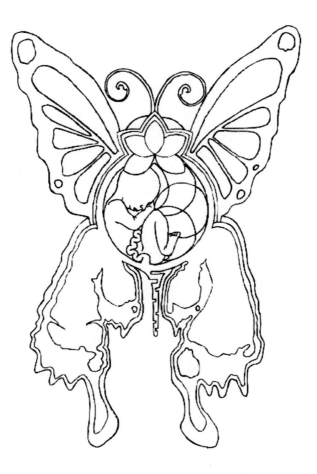

This Tattoo, was drawn by my son, Zion, for Jan Francisco, the midwife who received him into the world. She wears it between her shoulders. The lower part of the butterfly's wings are the footprints of her two lost children, Mikel and Chad, both born too soon. The five petals of the flower of life represent Jan's five living children.

After the death of a child, there are no easy answers, no recipes for survival. Everything is NOT fine. Living with this fact, as gracefully as one possibly can, is all there is.

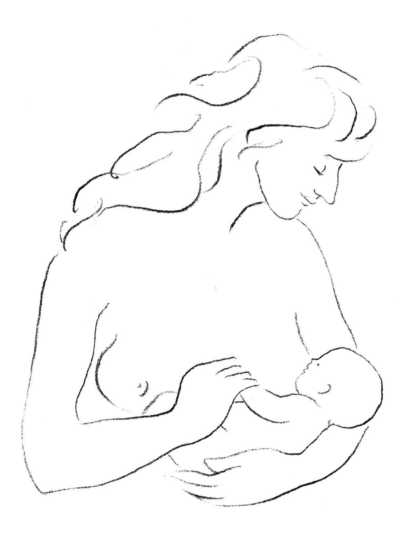

"Healing Birth Heals Mother Earth."

~ Jeannine Parvati... the Mother of BirthKeepers

Blossoming as an Organic Mother

To become a mother requires courage. One must have the faith necessary to allow an amazing and strange process to completely take over one's body and life. This is trust. This is bravery. This is the journey of the heroine. Heroism is the true nature of all women, everywhere on earth and for all times. For all women carry the potential of children, in their eggs. Making wise organic choices for your family means keeping your heart on a steady path. Don't beat yourself up, if you are not perfect, no one is. Being an organic mom does not mean you are against anything, it means you are gently and courageously for healthy choices, to benefit your family and our planet. So what if you snuck an ice cream, you remembered to bring your cloth bags to the market. Next time choose the healthy organic ice cream!

Perhaps the road to motherhood is treacherous and uncertain BECAUSE the job of motherhood has built into it, necessarily, the pre-requisite of heroism. From our experience of pregnancy, birth and postpartum we BECOME mothers. It is a powerful process of evolution. It is your personal mythical journey, a vision quest.

When we loose our power, and this happens in many ways to women; rape, the high rate of unnecessary cesarean birth, episiotomy, anesthetized birth, to name a few examples, the collective power of motherhood is diminished. When we are robbed we suffer a spiritual poverty, which takes time and nurturing to heal. Our mates, our children and society as a whole, suffer with us. Yet we mothers are still heroines, injured, scarred, too often not knowing our own virtue.

The prevailing message of modern civilization to pregnant women is; "You need medical assistance, pregnancy is pathology, it's too risky." "Give the responsibility to someone who knows what he is doing." "Let the experts take care of things." "Ask no questions." "Lie down, be quiet, birth in silent suffering." "Your womb is broken." Women who are abused medically leave the hospital with sadness and damaged self-esteem, instead of flying triumphantly into motherhood. Is it any wonder breastfeeding is on the decline and families are crumbling spiritually? This is the price we pay when we loose our natural power in the childbearing process.

You are NOT broken! As Ina May says: "Your body is not a lemon." The healthcare system is broken. We are all still striving to make Human Rights in Childbirth a possibility.

Every moment you spend now, as a pregnant woman, or new mother, enlightening yourself to your ecological birth and gentle mothering choices, is a bit of goodness won back into the world. The world your children will inherit and your daughters will bear children into. When families 'take back birth' we will witness a peaceful rEvolution of astounding beauty. Taking back Birth is a giant leap toward healing our Earth. Historians of the future will wonder, just why it took us so long to reclaim our human birthrights.

Yes, nearly every minute on Earth a mother dies of a complication of pregnancy or childbirth. Most of their deaths are preventable. Implementing Wisdom of nature's process is the necessary medicine that prevents maternal hemorrhage, and postnatal infection. Wisdom applied well lowers infant mortality. Wisdom cannot be replaced by technology, they must be employed together, wisely, along with our prayers. When we embrace our ancient wisdom, modern technology will serve us well. We will know when to use it, and when to let nature take her course. The wise marriage of Nature, Science and Prayer, reduces risk. Pregnancy is the journey toward wisdom. Learn from many teachers, but trust the teachers who BELIEVE in YOU, and inspire the awakening of your INNER KNOWING. Embrace the responsibility of being a wise woman. Don't let anyone take that away from you.

The Earth Mother is crying out under the strain of so much sorrow, pollution and injustice. She is our only home, our planet, and we face extinction, of our species and all species, if we do not awaken from this modern environmental nightmare. For this reason I am calling out for all humans to participate in Awakening Organic Birth.

There is no such thing as "safe" childbirth. There is childbirth in the context of wise choices, which differ depending upon life situation and environment, from woman to woman and baby to baby. In this book I encourage you to work in partnership with your BABY and your partner, midwife or doctor and doulas, to awaken your INNER KNOWING, your authentic self who will lead you to the most gentle, ecological, organic way you may birth, breastfeed and parent your child. With loving support, strength, and a good deal of courage, your personal path to motherhood, the way of the heroine, will become clear. Be wise beautiful natural mother.

Whisper to your Baby...

"May you live long enough to know why you were born."

~ Native American Blessing

Ibu Robin's Thanks Giving prayer:

Nurture your dream, love it as you would a newborn baby girl. Sometimes you will find your dream stays up all night
and cries for attention,
there is nothing to do, but give her attention.
Everyday, in some way, do something
toward the fulfillment of your dream.
Baby steps count, and they will get you where you need to go.
Your dream is your soul-mate, and deserves your love,
for collectively, the dreams of your generation will save our world.

Endnotes

1. Anne Grete Byskov, *Lancet,* 18 April 2002.

2. Gaur DS, Talekar M, Pathak VP (2007), "Effect of cigarette smoking on semen quality of infertile men", Singapore medical journal 48 (2): 119–23

3. Smartstork, gender selection

4. Why Skinny Moms Sometimes produce Fat Children AAAS Science news: http://news.sciencemag.org/2011/04/why-skinny-moms-sometimes-produce-fat-children accessed Sept 2015

5. Gian-Paolo Ravelli, M.D., M.S., Zena A. Stein, M.A., M.B., B.CH., and Mervyn W. Susser, M.B., B.CH., F.R.C.P. "Obesity in Young Men after Famine Exposure in Utero and Early Infancy" *N Engl J Med 1976;* 295:349-353 August 12, 1976 DOI: 10.1056/NEJM197608122950701 http://www.nejm.org/doi/pdf/10.1056/NEJM197608122950701 accessed Sept 2015

6. Premature Rupture of Membranes: Vaginal or Cesarean Delivery, *Healthline*

7. Robin Lim "Maternal Nutrition and Infant Feeding – Asking the Next Question" (Exerts from this writing were shared by Lim at the opening of the IFOAM 16th Organic World Congress, Modena, Italy, June 2008)

8. Dr. Inne Susante, *UNICEF Study on Maternal Mortalit*

9. Andrew Radford "The Ecological Impact of bottlefeeding", accessed on-line June 2016 http://abm.me.uk/wp-content/uploads/2012/10/Ecological-Impact-of-Bottlefeeding.pdf

10. Eligibility Requirements for Blood Donors: http://www.redcross-blood.org/donating-blood/eligibility-requirements

11. BMJ. 2011 Nov 15;343:d7157. doi: 10.1136/bmj.d7157.

12. Indian Pediatr. 2002 Feb;39(2):130-5.

13. JOURNAL OF TROPICAL PEDIATRICS, VOL. 58, NO. 6, 2012

14. The BMJ Effect of delayed versus early umbilical cord clamping on neonatal outcomes and iron status at 4 months: a randomised controlled trial http://www.bmj.com/content/343/bmj.d7157

15. J Perinat Neonat Nurs r Vo 2012, Rethinking Placental Transfusion and Cord Clamping Issues, Judith S. Mercer, PhD, CNM, FACNM, Debra A. Erickson-Owens, PhD, CNM

16. http://midwifethinking.com/2011/02/10/cord-blood-collection-confessions-of-a-vampire-midwife/

17. Why do obstetricians and midwives still rush to clamp the cord? BMJ 2010; BMJ 2010;341:c5447, http://www.bmj.com/rapid-response/2011/11/03/reis-it-time-end-early-cord-clamping

18. http://midwifethinking.com/2011/02/10/cord-blood-collection-confessions-of-a-vampire-midwife/

19. Die Wahrscheinlichkeit, dass ein Mensch im Laufe seines Lebens überhaupt eine Stammzelltransplantation (egal ob aus Nabelschnurblut oder Knochenmark) braucht, schätzt die Uniklinik in Heidelberg auf 0,06% bis 0,46% abhängig vom Lebensalter, das erreicht wird. Entsprechend gering ist die Wahrscheinlichkeit, dass bei einer Transplantion das eigene Nabelschnurblut verwendet wird: Die Schätzungen reichen von einer Wahrscheinlichkeit von 1:1400 bis 1:200.000. http://www.babycenter.de/a36661/warum-ist-nabelschnurbluteinlagerung-umstritten#ixzz3EKUNPq4X

20. http://www.whale.to/a/morley17.html

21. Hubungan penundaan pengkleman tali pusat dengan peningkatan kadar hemoglobin, hematokrit dan bilirubin pada neonatus yang lahir dari ibu anemia, oleh: I Gusti Ayu Mirah Widhi Sastri, NPM: 131020090046, tesis Program Pascasarjana Universitas Padjadjaran 2012.

22. Neonatal Resuscitation (LifeStart) http://www.inditherm.co.uk/medical/neonatal-resuscitation-lifestart/

23. http://www.epistemonikos.org/de/documents/e068abb1a37d6f4c343068377945144da56c483f?doc_lang=en - Late umbilical cord-clamping as an intervention for reducing iron deficiency anemia in term infants in developing and industrialized countries: a systematic review.

24. 100+ circumcision deaths each year in United States http://www.circinfo.org/USA_deaths.html sourced 5 July, 2016

25. Van Howe RS. A cost-utility analysis of neonatal circumcision. Med Decis Making. 2004;24:584-601.

26. CIRP. Medical organization official policy statements. Available online at: http://www.cirp.org/library/statements/

27. Anand KJS, for the International Evidence-Based Group for Neonatal Pain. Consensus statement for the prevention and management of pain in the newborn. Arch Pediatr Adolesc Med. 2001;155:173-80.